BECOMING THE CHAMPION

VOLUME 1: AWARENESS

KOREY CARPENTER

DAWN PUBLISHING

© 2020 Korey Carpenter

Published by Dawn Publishing
www.dawnbates.com
The moral right of the author has been asserted.

For quantity sales or media enquiries, please contact the publisher at the website address above.

Cataloguing-in-Publication entry is available from the British Library.

ISBN: 978-0-9957322-8-5 (paperback)
978-0-9957322-9-2 (ebook)

All rights reserved. No part of this book may be reproduced, stored in a retrieval system, communicated or transmitted in any form or by means without written permission. All inquiries should be made to the publisher at the above address.

Disclaimer: The material in this publication is of the nature of general comment only and does not represent professional advice. It is not intended to provide specific guidance for particular circumstances and should not be relied on as the basis for any decision to take action or not to take action on any matters which it covers.

CONTENTS

Foreword   v
Gratitude   ix
Introduction   xi

1. An invitation   1
2. Point of the Story   7
3. My Story   11
4. The flame ignites the phoenix   19
5. Strike One   23
6. Sharpening the tools   27
7. Left to the wolves   31
8. Raging fire   35
9. 3rd Eye Open   39
10. The Initiation   49
11. The Hunters Moon   55
12. Birthday Reality   63
13. They are real if you are open to it   67
14. Christmas Surprise   71
15. Screaming Blood   75
16. The Cabins   81
17. The Cabins Door Buster   105
18. Your Decision to control your mind   109
19. The Woods   113
20. Pumpkin Center   129

Author Note   141
About the Author   143

FOREWORD

'Growing up is hard to do', a great songwriter once wrote.

'School days are the happiest days of your life', apparently.

The first statement is so very true for a great number of people, for a vast array of reasons. Whilst we may know what is going on in our own lives, and those we know, love and care about; the lives of those in our local communities, countries and neighboring continents is just something very few of us give a second thought to.

We are so wrapped up in our own lives and challenges that it takes something so profoundly upsetting or disturbing to bring our attention to something much more sinister and upsetting to wake us up from our slumber of indifference.

Being woken up can come from a multitude of places. A docufilm, our travels, news footage, or meeting someone who has lived and grown up in a set of circumstances which are so alien to us, and so horrifying that we cannot begin to process what life must have been like for them.

Depending on how we meet this person, and how they have chosen to live their life will of course depend on how we interact with them. Some will have not had the resources, the awakening or the capacity to overcome some of the most horrendous acts of violence and abuse known to humans.

Some will have had that knowing deep down inside that they were always born for more, that they were born to serve through the suffering, rise through the trauma to bring awareness and healing to others, as well as bring about social change. Korey Carpenter is one such individual.

What you are about to read, not just in this book but the ones which follow, will open your eyes to aspects of society which you probably thought you were a million miles away from; even if you believe in the six degrees of separation.

Getting to know Korey, his journey and his passion to make a difference in this world has been an emotional rollercoaster. As a mother my heart broke for him and those children in his community. As a woman I felt numb for a variety of reasons. As a leader of humanity, an activist for social change the fire within me erupted. As Korey's coach, mentor and soul sister, I am in awe of the man he has become, the passion he has for healing others, and for the courage he is owning, and sharing, with you all.

It takes a very brave person to face up to traumas and pain from their past, choosing to go on to heal from the wounds caused by said traumas. For that person to then step up and share their journey with others so society can learn the real truths of what goes on behind closed doors, takes a depth of courage not many have. To then choose to take on society, to awaken and heal individuals on a global stage… that takes a champion; and Korey is a champion on so many levels.

With his story, his courses and his coaching, not to mention his media appearances, he is changing society and exposing those who consciously choose to look the other way whilst others inflict pain and suffering on others.

His story is not for the feint hearted, nor is it a pleasant read in places. With his Southern accent and his kindness coming through in his words, you will hear how the darkness of child abuse, drugs, violence and the blind eye of society has not made him a 'statistic' but a champion of the people, a champion of men, and a role model for men everywhere.

Korey, it is an honour to know you, to walk this path with you and to watch you defend your title as champion each and every single day.

May the world know your name, and may your words inspire social change and strength in those who need it the most.

With love always,

Dawn

Dawn Bates
Author, Coach, Strategist, Publisher
www.dawnbates.com

GRATITUDE

The people that deserve the first THANK YOU in the writing of this book are those who first believed in me and my potential.

For sticking with me, supporting my vision, and your creative nature thanks for being my best friend and wife, Ani.

For all your love, support, and confidence in me, thank you my amazing soul family, you know who you are. Thank you all for choosing me as your family.

For all the time and work devoted, the coaching and developing, and for being awesome, a big thank you to my coach and publisher, Dawn Bates.

Most importantly, thank you God Source, for the journey that has been my life and to my parents.

Without my journey I would not be creating this book, become a healer, nor have the opportunity to lead others to Becoming the Champion.

INTRODUCTION

This is my personal story of becoming the champion of my own life. No matter your story, we all have the same one because we all have experienced some degree of trauma in our life which we allowed to shape us. Most often we are shaped to accepting the role of a victim in a traumatic situation. I felt like a victim of bad circumstances, bad people, and unfair predispositions the majority of my life. But being a victim of circumstance is how you give away your power. When you feel powerless, you wait and hope for circumstance (the very thing to which you surrendered power) to change or save you.

I am here to tell you the one that can save you or change your situation is you. You must become the champion that goes back and saves you from being the victim. This is the very process that created the 'champion'. You may have heard of being your highest version or your higher self. After embarking on my own mindset and healing journey I realized that every trauma healed, every blockage removed, and every choice made to rewire felt like winning! Soon it came to me... the highest self is a champion. And not just any champion but me as the champion.

So, when do you become the champion?

The thing about a champion is that the title always needs defending.

The title will need defending through every 'round' of life. Throughout this book, you will be guided to relating types of trauma and resetting them in your timeline to take back your power and lock in your win.

ONE
AN INVITATION

Have you ever been in a situation where you know this is not the way you want to live your life?

Have you thought to yourself, *I do not want to do this anymore?*

Something about how your life, and the people you find yourself being around, is not what you genuinely want out of life?

Well, I think at some point in our life, we have all been there. These points are the moments we choose one of those 360 different choices.

Now some paths may seem to start out like the one you see yourself finishing but forgot that every moment along the path, you have a choice to make. One distraction can lead you off the path you started by not stay grounded and connected.

Pay more attention to the path you are walking, because one misstep off the path can lead you astray.

Blockages and traumas are conditioning that keeps you afraid of the dark. Simply put, the fears you keep in your subconscious mind and think about as you react from a state of fear.

This is how you have been taught, shown, or behave. These blockages can hold you back, keeping you from succeeding and reaching your highest potential. Your mind and body working together to unite and balance with your soul.

You will not fail at anything you are working to receive when serving your best service to the world; what your human design was meant to do whilst here and during this experience.

Each of us can do something better than others, and we all need to be a part of the team that helps make change for the service to all. Not one person is to do it all. We are meant to do things together, and together we can do anything. Each one of us are a part of some team somewhere and if each one of you did what you are best at, we would solve all problems that we would face together.

To be ready to open to the next level you must be all in and make sure you are ready for this. Stepping into your next up level is one of rewiring and letting go of the old ego. If you are not happy with the version of yourself you are right now, how will you know the version you want will be enough?

Please write it down and go into detail with what you want to be.

If you need more time, mark it down and come back to it later when you have time.

Now let us look at what I would suggest doing as we go through this story of my past. I only wish to share it because it is mine to share. I know it will help others to see what blockages I have overcome and how my blockages were formed.

I invite you to investigate what challenges you, confronts you and the reason why. How can you become the champion in these moments of being challenged and confronted?

Try to look as I do and see if you are ready to release. You are never 'wrong' or 'too late' to release and remove old patterns. You must let them surface and sometimes you must feel the pain to release it.

If something is coming up, then you need to dump it out and refill your cup with what you want.

There is a way to dig up and remove all blockages. If there are layers you can work them out in stages.

Blockages caused by a trauma will need more work to remove a deeper wound programmed in your nervous system.

If you want to know about blockages look at your patterns. The pattern of winning, losing or getting along, there is a pattern you are living through. Your taught skills and learned habits are picked up along the way. If you are not happy, then you are not happy with something in your life, and things keep happening no matter how many times you try. There is this pattern of choices and decisions you make that might keep circling back over and over. Something you say, like "this always happens to me" or "of course that did not work out for me". Phrases you say about how your life is somehow vexed. These are taught and can be removed and can be reprogrammed to your natural state, the "happy, energetic and loving to everyone around you" state of being.

Spotting the repeated phrases you speak and identifying the patterns to see how you can pull out your own triggers and view life from a grounded honest version of who you are, and who you are meant to be during this human experience. By you living in your truth and doing what you love most, you will be able to serve at the highest of your potential while helping the ones around you to live a better happier life.

When you amplify your love and energy, you will raise the energy and love for the ones with the same blood. You will see how, when you do what you love and be who you are, you will attract the people who are supposed to be in your life. The people who try to hold you down will just disappear when you are in balance.

There are so many different types of patterns and blockages. The main ones will be religious and family beliefs that get pushed on to you. These can be distorted and sometimes misunderstood. You must be able to see the blockage from more angles than just yours and truly go back into the moment. Allow things to surface and say, "Okay, this happened," and then you can request from your subconscious to remove all negative emotions from the memory. You gave all the energy to the memory and logged it away with pain or fear, and therefore the body reacts in all the many ways it knows how. Self-sabotage, doubt, envy, greed, jealousy, or trying to live someone else's life. Being a version of yourself that someone else made you into. That is not living, and being who you are for only yourself, so you can be the best version of you for the ones closest to you will benefit the most.

You will succeed at whatever you take on, and genuinely want to do with your life, and fulfil all your desires and dreams. You will have everything you want, when you see and remove blockages that are keeping you from attracting abundance and wealth.

The most and deepest blockages come from your youth and from an age we barely remember. This is a place where you need time to yourself to go deep.

Log memories and write them down. I find it helps to physically get it out on paper.

Just keep in mind, when something is telling you, *I think it is like (XYZ)*, look at the belief and see if that something is what you were taught or something you believe because of an experience?

Look for the connections and feel into why.

Be honest and real and you will know the answer.

Our life begins in the first moments we can retain information and logging emotions and feelings. We forget emotions can override our thoughts, and our thoughts can trigger emotions. There is a way to acknowledge and know what is right and let go of whatever is stopping you from letting go.

Take that next step and open the door. You are only waiting for yourself. You control you, and your emotions are due to how you react in that moment. Each decision you make and step you take will be the path to choose.

To get back on track and find your way is to feel into every decision. Even if your choice does not work out, there is a lesson to learn and to share so others do not make them. Learn from each other, and if you love someone, be honest about what you feel.

The best thing we can all do is accept that we are all so different but also the same.

Just think of the steps it takes to create you here right now. The planet you are on and the life we all share is so special and delicate to be honest. Find yourself where you are and move forward from there. Take the next best steps you feel are right and what makes you feel good about moving forward. What can you do to make the changes you feel you want? Where do you need to go and find the information? Who can you talk to?

How to take the first step forward? Take the time you need to make the right decisions by feeling into every choice. If it feels right and you know it in your soul, then step in that direction. If you need time to think and cannot see a way. Close your eyes and focus on your heart. The answers will come to you once you have truly and fully opened you heart to the answers.

TWO
POINT OF THE STORY

Leading others to dig into their own. When you listen to someone's story you have quick memories go by and you never take time remembering why you have that memory?

What energy do you harbor, and feelings do you have towards the memories you have?

When you read it, you can take more time to get deeper into you own memories. You can stop and take notes and bullet point moments you can relate to as you read at your own pace and in your own time.

Each memory attached to the program we have learned and have been taught by others who did not know better.

The times and systems have changed, and we must grow with the evolution of life and the change in how we live our lives. There is a point that our parents are no longer the teacher. It comes to a point when we become the teachers of the teachers.

If your parents do not stay up with technology and what is moving forward in the times and how society has been changed. They raised us during different times and every 10 years the world changes. Remove your blockages of what you learned form a generation who did not have the support we have now. The free access to information where we can learn about anything.

We must teach if you do not know the answer you need to go to where you can get the information. If you need to help your children learn you should learn it too; so, you can be there to support them if they need help.

I know you do not have the time, and I get it, all my brothers and sister have kids and I hear and see it firsthand. Have you ever thought that if your child saw you doing extra to help them learn, they too would feel the love and put even more effort in to doing better? The time you would have together learning and helping one another is precious, it builds a strong bond between you and the shared experience will never be lost. Just showing honest support to do better and letting them know they will succeed if they continue to try. You only fail if you have given up and stop trying.

If you want to truly step up and do what you love and live life with enjoyment an abundance you need to know what you want. Why you are here, and what it is you are to do? If you do not love your job and want to be happy about what you are doing. Then see what is holding you back and remove it. If you are not able to find the partner you desire, you only must-see what blockages you have and remove them. You can reset your whole design and re-program to work at your optimal peak. If you are happy and balanced while doing what you love the love will flow back to you and the ones closets to you. If you want to help, make you and anyone in your life happy all you must do is be the happiest you can be by removing anything keeping you from feeling it. If you can feel as if you are living in the here and now and can see what all is available and how to keep track of your path. All it takes after you have removed blockages and start to move forward. You will have a better knowing of how to remove them for yourself and for other you want to help. There will be triggers and layers that come and go. When you can recognize the pattern of your old habit you will get to a point of reacting to it and releasing it quicker as you go. Allow for your old habit to be just a reminder or once upon a time ago. It is just a story of a way that happened a time ago. Give no negative energy to having the feelings and sometimes needing time to let things go. Years and years of burying pain and emotions take time to reset and heal from. Breathing is extremely helpful and smiling to. Move your energy around and make sure you are ready to make the change of only your ego.

Why My Story? It is just that. My story. So instead of making one up I will use mine as the example and then I can explain the blockages and traumas I worked through. This will help you to relate and to see what comes up for you while we work through your blockages. Going back thousands of years we would learn by telling stories. We would tell tales and magical spells and stories lived like flesh and bone. How kings and wives and brothers of all kinds would love and kill one another. The way we related and shared our information we would work together and would establish a thrown. We would rise together and love one another until greed would turn brother against brother. The moment we stop caring about the others around us is the moment we fail as a people. We only have each other to help one another to move forward teaching the next generation. We have lost the times when we lived as a tribe and worked for the community. Life taken over with distractions and cover of the truth of what you are capable of. My story will help you think about yours and I say if you have a special friend or a spouse to do this with, it can really help a friend or a loved one to go through this together. It helps with the company to keep on track and not let the story run and get you off track. The human species is a tribal one and likes to have others around. Maybe not a lot but in our natural state we are happiest when surrounded by love. So, to read through each story and see what comes up. I would write it down and continue or dig deeper if you feel too and to work through and see what comes up. Again, this is at you our pace and in your own time. If you try to rush it, you will not dig deep enough and if you do not do it. You probably need some time to get things sorted but this will be here when you are ready.

I will tell the story and show you how to look from outside without judgment and realize what you need to so you can release from the attachment. Learn the lessons and be thankful you can pass on the teaching to others as you remove your own. You will see the more you remove the more that you can help the others. Friends and family will start to have luck and you will attract what you want with abundance and the energy to do what you want to do. Your flow state will be easy to access, and you will be able to be in your bliss and happy balanced state of mind. The darkest moments in our lives can help others to see the light in their own. By helping each other you can also heal your own wounds by giving what hurt you a good purpose. Positive energy will heal the deepest wound. Being witnessed and supported will empower the process and help to speed up the healing. Love from another and a gift of love in return can change the weather. Love light exchanged and cycled like water reconnect to your heart center and refill your cup with love water. Flush out the old and spritz up the new. Share your authentic version of you. Tell your own story and how you removed your blockages as well. Not everyone will relate but to the ones who are meant to will be called and come to learn and share what they are going through. Look at each memory to see what emotions you hold on to. What images you relate emotions to and your ideas and opinions of others. Really see yourself for who you and who you want to be. Then see what is keeping you from embodying that.

THREE
MY STORY

Mine started when I was four years young. I remember watching Scooby-Doo on TV and playing in a large yard. Mother, Father, Brother and two Sisters. I remember family times cooking out playing and having fun. Faded memories of a big family and so many smiles I remember seeing from so long ago. A storm shaking the trailer and breaking a window. Running down the hall and a cat named Murphy attacking my legs and taking me to the floor. I would laugh and play and wrestle with my father smelling of oil and diesel fuel. Moved into a bigger house with a room full of toys and a TV with cartoons. Thunderstorms would scare me from the feel of the thunder. So exciting and so thrilling I liked how I felt after. There was family that lived behind us and close to town and I had so much to play with. My dad built a sand box covered by a porch a slide attached and swings. I remember putting my hand in concrete on the front porch and playing in the sprinkler running out front. Riding a bicycle with training wheels and falling just once. The times I was sitting in my father's Pontiac Trans AM with a Phoenix on the hood. I loved looking at the lights on the dash while my sister held me. My father's daughter from another than my mother but still family to me. My uncle picking me up by my ears like he was when he was young like me. Country fields sometimes covered with snow. Simple yet loving and I was comfortable and felt safe where I was. The funny little stories of my years as a boy flirting with girls in the store. Running in the yard barefoot and loving the way it felt. Laughing with family happy to be and so many hugs I remember.

Then one day, my mother packed everything in the house into a big yellow box truck, put me in the middle of the seats where there was a sliding door and a mattress on the floor in the box and everything else packed in behind us. I was told to sit down or go to sleep. I had no idea what was going on or where we were going but I was simply happy to go for a ride and felt like she made me my brother and sister a fort inside this big truck. As we left the area, I heard my mother say, "Oh shit! There he is," as I looked over the dashboard and seen my father's Pontiac Trans AM with a phoenix on the hood go by.

"There's Dad!" I said and popped up excited to see him go by.

My mother smacked me and said, "Sit down and shut up. Get back there and hold still."

I had no idea what was going on. I had no idea that would be the last image I would see of my father for a long time. As days went by the questions I would ask where not answered I realized my mother really did not like me asking and getting up front to see what was going on. My brother and sister could move about and sit up front, but I had to sit still, shut up, be quiet, stop moving, stop asking questions, just go to sleep. I never spent a lot of time with her and come to think of it, I started to notice my presence would anger her or she just did not want to talk to me. The time we actually spent together was less than anyone else I was around. She was there, but the others were her children, and I was just the baby.

My sister never liked me from what I can recall, and my older brother acted like I did not exist. So, to occupy myself I would have to create games and try to self-entertain. Talking to my self and trying to see where we were going the best I could.

One day I was in the back of the truck trying to sleep and I heard my mother say, "Stay still and be quiet." Closing the door to the front leaving us kids in the back with no air in the heat. She pulled the truck over on the side of the road and stopped. I could hear someone walk alongside the truck outside and start talking to my mother. My sister told me to shut up and stay still. After a little bit of time she started the truck and continued down the road. Opening the door, I found out she was pulled over for speeding and lied to the officer so he would not give her a ticket, happy and bragging about what she did.

The landscape looks so different then to what I'd seen at the house we lived in with my father. This beautiful red and brown landscape speckled with green bushes and huge mountains off in the distance. I was mesmerized by its never-ending horizon.

One day my mother pulled over and picked up a hitchhiker and spoke to him like she knew him. He was a large man, very dirty and had scruffy hair. The biggest hands I have ever seen and blond hair covering his body. Tanned by the sun, and his loud voice was intimidating. His energy was like a kid. My mother went on about what she was doing and where we were going, but I still had no idea what was going on.

Once he noticed me, he asked who I was.

She replied, "Korey my youngest."

He looked at me, then at her and said, "Who does he belong to?"

She replied, "It is a long story."

I will never forget his face and the look he gave me. I could see in his eyes the look that he knew something I did not, and he was playing the story in his mind. The grin he had, and how his eyes looked down, I could see in his reaction. He turned to the front and started back up about where he was heading.

Shortly after that they were talking about what he has been doing a spoke of getting out of a place called prison and he was walking back home. My mother told him he was crazy trying to walk two states and how dangerous it was to do that. The man laughed and pulled out a gun that looked like Yosemite Sam's from the looney tunes I remember seeing on TV. She told him to put that away and asked him what he was doing with that?

My mother said, "If you get caught with that, you will go back for life."

The man replied, "I have no intentions on going back, and if they try, they will have to kill me." He opened the round chamber and pulled out one of the bullets and showed it to me. He said, "This right here will kill a cop with one shot."

My mother told the man he was crazy and told him to put it away. The man took the bullet out of my hand, loaded the gun rolled down the window and shot a hole in a sign going down the road in the middle of the day. No time to plan just pure reaction he was loaded and off he goes. The smile I remember, as he took aim and I had no idea what was about to happen.

I fell back from the concussion holding my head and could not hear. All I could see is my mother screaming at him as he was laughing. If I close my eyes, I can still feel the trauma from all those years ago. The throbbing and the pain I felt in my head to the sound of solid hit to a bell. It was not of fear or just the pain that I felt. It was from the shock of the unknown power the gun.

After I realized I was not hurt physically but my emotions overwhelmed me, I was able to stop crying and sit up. He told me that I was okay and sorry he did not tell me to cover my ears. He put the gun away and had a smile from ear to ear. I could see in his mind he was ready to use the gun on anyone who challenged his choices. He was an outlaw of the west and he would die in a way he would choose and needed no one's approval. Only now I realize he was a man of many wounds and hated himself so much he was ready to move on from this world. I was able to see inside his heart and I could feel what his smile was hiding. I never seen him again after stopping to get fuel in a small town and he decided that is where he wanted to go.

After getting back on the road I remember thinking about what he would do where would he go and what he would become? My mind started to wonder in way it had not before. I started looking at people more and more and tuning into what I could feel how they feel. Really looking at someone else with open curiosity I could start to see visions of what they felt or what their life was like. I did not understand it at the time, but I would run wild with visions and feelings from being around others. I never thought I was right, but I was open to other's experiences. Every time we would stop to get fuel or food, I was unable to control the flood of information I was seeing. In my mind's eye and the feelings, I would feel for the visions I would receive. My mother was full of pain and fear. My brother and sister in the truck was very dull and quiet. My brothers mind was one that processes more information than I could keep up with. While my sister was in the clouds thinking of the most random things as they would come in. I became a watcher of others and learned to tune in without trying.

Once we made it to a town surrounded by tall trees and mountains in the distance. I learned that we had to move into a small apartment. I could feel it was a place of pain and suffering. I did not like it and would ask my mother where my dad was and if he was on the way. She would tell me to shut up and go to my room that I had to share with my brother and sister. Three kids in one small room and neither my brother nor my sister wanted me around. I was placed in this new place with no one and nothing that felt familiar, nor any kind of happiness. I would create my own games and would have to play games with myself and create friends in my mind. I would talk to trees, bushes, large rocks or boulders, and my shadow. People would see this and judge me, telling me I was a weird little kid or that I was crazy. So, I would look for something to do away from others so people would stop being mean to me. I could see how they felt towards me while calling me these names and the judgment they would place in their minds. I separated from the people that I was around, and never did my mother, brother, or sister want me around.

I never felt that I did anything wrong, but I did know and could feel that they did not want me around. I could feel the disgusted feeling my mother would feel when she looked at me, and the hate my sister would stare at me with. My brother never gave me much thought and treated me like a puppy that he would talk to if I were in the way, and would tell me what not to touch or play with something, especially if it was his. I spent most my time outside and alone trying to make friends, but every time I would try, I was told that they are not allowed to talk to me. I did not understand why I was cast aside and why no one ever wanted to play or hang out. I did not have many toys or things I could call my own, so I would play games like how high I could climb or how fast could I run from one side of the parking lot to the other. Then a few days later everything changed.

I remember one night while sitting in the room with my brother and sister I could hear my mother talking to a man in the living room. I peeked out and I could see my mother sitting at the table across from a tall man. She was hunched down and looking at the table like if she was in trouble for doing something wrong. I could feel the shame and disappointment in how much she hated herself at that moment. I wanted to run over and hug her and protect her from feeling how I felt looking at her. Then the tall man looked over at me and I will never forget the look on his face and the pain I felt made me want to pass out. I felt dizzy and like I wanted to fall over. He then had a slight grin and turned towards me and waved his large hands for me to come over to him. Curiously, I slowly walked over as my mother would not look at me. As I got closer, I could feel his energy change. The pain he felt he pushed down, and he smiled bigger as I got closer. The man picked me up, set me on his leg, put his arm around my side and patted me on my left thigh and said, "Hello son."

I smiled back and said, "Hi."

I could feel his heart and the love this large man held in his chest. I felt safe and accepted for the first time since my father. I did not understand the look on my mother's face. Not until later in life would I find out why and how I was to this man. He smelled like beer and cigarettes and smiled and seemed happy to meet me.

Not fully understanding the full dynamic of the situation, I went on my way and off to bed. The next day I did not see that man again and was told that he was my brother and sisters' father. I did not know at the time they had a different father and I did not understand how that happened. When I would ask, I would get told that I am a bastard child and have no father. I was confused and I would tell people I have a father and would ask what is a bastard? The response was always the same. You are. So, for a while I would introduce myself as Korey the bastard child of my mother. People would give me the strangest looks and ask why I would say that? I would explain that is what my family tells me I am. The looks and the feelings made me upset for I did not know what they meant or why they would look and feel the way I would feel when I engaged in conversation. All I wanted was to meet new people and have friends to spend time with. I did not want to be alone but no one in town or in the area we lived in wanted to be my friend. I felt something was wrong with me and wanted to change who I was. I was alone some of the time and would wish to see my father. I did not understand why he was not coming and why my mother would not let me call him. The people I started to meet kept me at a distance and people seemed to not know what to do with me or if to talk to me. Like there was something wrong with me and no one will tell what it is.

I want to know why I was here and what I was supposed to do and if I had any purpose. I wished at night to take off and fly back to my father where I felt safe and loved. Waking in this place every day and all I wanted to do was wake up back with my dad and apparently, I had a different life to survive.

FOUR
THE FLAME IGNITES THE PHOENIX

One day a man came home with my mother and they were kissing and rubbing on each other in the living room and I asked who he was. They told me to go to my room and shut the door and to not come out. Days went by and he never left. My brother and sister went to school, and I had to wait until I was old enough to go.

He would watch TV, drink, smoke, and make phone calls all day. He had other men come over while my mother was at work and they would pick on me while I was in the apartment. I was fascinated by the matches they would use to light the things they smoked and hated the smell it made. I did not like it when they would get in my face and tell me to leave or go somewhere until the streetlights came on. The smell of their breath from the beer they would drink. The look on their face as they would call me a punk or little bitch for asking for anything. He would flinch at me like he was going to hit me if I ever bothered him or his friends.

I could feel the hate and started to see a very dark shadow forming around his whole body. Not like a glow but a dark outline surrounding him. There was a lot I was feeling and the way he would look at me made me feel uncomfortable. When he would smile it would make the hair on the back of my neck stand straight up and I did not like looking at him. He was very loud, and he would never ask for anything. He would just take and eat my food or go through whatever he wanted in the kitchen. If I told him that it was for me, my brother, or sister, he would tell me to shut the fuck up and go away. I did not like him touching my mother and would grab her chest and butt in front of us kids and the actions they would perform in the living room was not what any child should see or have to hear. The sounds and the things he would say to her I did not understand but I know I felt so angry he was even touching her.

(Blockage) This was one of the first blockages I can remember. I found this to be the reason that I have the reaction I do to all males who try for any female I have in my life that I care about. No not like or want to be with, but the ones I have love for, like family or kin. I would always size up any man that wanted to court or talk to anyone I deemed under my protection. Also, another part of it was I always felt I needed to protect any girl or females that I had around because of the blockage from seeing this kind of action as a four-year-old boy. It was from wanting to protect my mother from the low vibe man I seen her with, and how he treated her and us kids was not okay with me.

I had this deep knowing that he was bad and not what I wanted for my mother. My father was all I wanted to see her with and if I ever said anything about it, she would get mad at me and tell me how my father did not want me and wanted an abortion. I had no idea what that was, but I did know I wanted this man out of our life and away from my mother.

This will cause any child to reject any other for their parent. I do not care mom or dad. If you are a child of separated parents, you need to look at the feelings you had towards the situation. It will show you if you have negative response to anyone you care about in life when they bring a new partner around. This is a reaction from a childhood blockage. No one else is good enough for who it is you care about and have love for. They will never be enough for them if you do not remove the blockage and accept this is just part of their life and journey.

I was always told to "sit over there" or to "go away" and I was never allowed to be involved and no one would ever show me or teach me anything. I did not have any friends and was not allowed to go out or sit, but also never allowed to be in the house with other people.

I was told to be seen from a distance and never heard. If I asked a question, they would smack me or shove me away.

I would ask for water or something to eat, and they would tell me to figure it out or starve. I had to learn to make things on my own and if I made a mess and did not clean it up immediately, they would punish me like it was a game. These men would push me and call me names and though I did not know what these names meant I knew they were mean by the tone of the voice they would use.

Each friend that would come over or stop by would act the same and did not like me being in the apartment while they were there. Some of his friends was not allowed to be around children and I was told to go outside while they were there. Later finding out he did something to his stepdaughter and by law was not allowed around kids.

These monsters and animals who I was to learn from, watching and listening to how they would plan robberies, and talk about what they would do to these girls and women in the neighborhood. They would laugh and joke about killing police and what they wanted to do to the men in government. They would talk about other men who owed them money and would go into detail on how they were going to kill them and make them watch as they raped their wife's. The smiles and grins on their faces as they would talk about the things they lived for.

Reflection

This would lead me to see that I have a deep disrespect for men who talk like they are violent and hateful. Men needing to be monsters and act so violent are only hiding from the truth that they are afraid of others seeing them in their true light. I would later in life have issues and challenge these men and was the reason I was so violent as a child and young adult. I was always looking for the biggest of bad man around and if he would not stand with me, he would be placed as against me.

I learned to walk and talk like a killer and would put fear into others by my actions. Some would try to fight, and I had to know when to walk away so I did not go to prison for murdering a boy trying to be a man. These are the lessons and programs other men who choose to be around lesser men will do. They want nothing new and refuse to meet new people. I see this as a blockage of not wanting to ever face the man they fear. Scared boys not wanting to be tested and afraid of others seeing them as they truly are. I was ready to die and thought of dying in battle as honorable, and as all men should. This is a filter of hate and ignorance that is learned from another and taught by someone who was treated in such a way. This template would be fueled by anger and rage covered by pain and sadness. These angry men and boys only need to know they can choose and if they don't want to be like the ones who did what they did to them, they have to choose to be who they truly are and that it is okay to be the way they are meant to be. What others teach you and tell you that you are not what they will never be does not have to be the truth if you choose to be yourself and find your own way.

FIVE
STRIKE ONE

One day, my mother's boyfriend and several friends locked them self into my mothers' room and where doing something I was not allowed to see. They did this often and I knew it would be enough time for me to be out of my room and try to see if there was other kids to try to play with or I would play games by myself.

One of his friends left his pack of matches out on the table and I wanted to strike one to see how they worked. I was fascinated by them when I would watch them light it to light their cigarettes or whatever it was they were smoking.

I went into my room and pulled one match off the pack and struck it across the strip igniting a flam. I stared with amazement and as it got to my finger it burned me, so I dropped it and I landed between the wall and my mattress. My finger hurt so I ran to the bathroom and ran cold water over my hand to cool it.

As I walked out of the bathroom the fire alarm went off and I looked in my room to see the mattress on fire and smoke running up the wall. They ran out of the room screaming at me and grabbing bowls and cups of water putting out the flames. As the fire department and sheriff came and questioned the reason, they also found out one of my mother's friend had something he was in trouble for and was arrested. After everyone left and the fire was out I got the first beating of my life and will never forget the feeling of being thrown into a wall, smacked to the ground, kicked in the stomach, grabbed by the throat and told that he was going to kill me for bringing the police to the apartment.

The next day while everyone was gone, I tried to stay away from him, and he was in the living room. He told me to get out and go somewhere. He didn't want to look at me or see me for the whole day. As I walked by looking at the ground, he said just keep walking until I see water. I looked at him and asked why? From me questioning him he jumped up snatched me up slammed me against the wall and told me to shut the fuck up and do not question him. Crying from the fear of him he said I'll give you something to cry about and I'm going to teach you a lesson about playing with fire. He grabbed me by the wrist and held my hand open while he took out a yellow lighter and burned the palm of my left hand with the flame. As I was screaming, I could see the excitement and thrill he was getting out of hurting me and causing this kind of pain. I fell to the floor screaming and if I tried to close my hand it hurt so I had to hold it open and was blowing on it. He yelled at me to stop screaming like a bitch and kicked me in the back. He said get out and went back to the couch like nothing happened. I ran outside to the nearest creek and dipped my hand in the water. Blessed I was there was a creek with mineral water to help ease the pain. As I sat there holding my hand underwater the images of his face and the feelings, he was having from what he did to me played over and over.

Days went by and all I could do was try to stay away, and to myself. My mother was mad I caught the bed on fire. My brother and sister felt the same. This man pushed me and smacked me every day after. Making me do pushups until my arms gave out. Sit ups until I could not move. Hold the push up position with his foot on my back pushing me down. Telling me I am unwanted and hated. A bastard child who should just run away or how he would wish I would get snatched and taken.

If my mother tried to tell them to stop, she would also get a punishment of some sort. He would grab her by the throat and push her down. So, to try to protect her, I would never tell her what he did to me so she would not get the same as I did. My brother and sister were lucky they had school to go to. I could not wait to go to school so I was able to get away from this monster.

I would sit back and listen to everyone around me and how they would steal and take from others and what they would do after they would rob from men and women at gun point or with a knife. I could see the excitement and thrill they would get bragging about the kind of monsters they are and what else they were to go do.

Reflection

Never feeling wanted or worthy of love. Always feel like an outcast and no one wants me around. My life meant nothing to the people I would have to be around.

Later in life all my decisions would be well thought out from the fear of being wrong. Over analyze everything and cut off all emotions to my mother and other feminine energy in my life.

I would look at other women that reminded me of my mother. I would grow to have hate for their existence and have no pity or love for the connection to my mother. Everyone around me was also blind to me and how I felt.

Therefore, I never had relationships, and when I did, I was not the best to be around when you needed cuddles or when you would cry for 'no reason'. Sometime girls need to release, and I did not know that is one of the ways they are able to do so.

This blockage created a way for me to control my emotions, and judge others for the life they were crying about. It was not as bad as the young girls around me had it, so I would treat them like weak scared little girls, instead of being there for them holding space as needed.

I had hatred for the feminine energy, because the one who gave me life acted as if she did not care if I were to die or be killed. Without addressing it, the problem would grow and dig deeper and deeper; as the story goes, burying it under layer after layer of what I would harbor in feelings and hate.

Another blockage from this would be not opening to new people and shutting my emotions off not allowing love form other sources. When others would try to show me love I would shut it down by spitting on it or rejecting it. No, I don't need you blah blah blah. This was the way I started living and surviving.

SIX
SHARPENING THE TOOLS

Some of the friends that came over would show me their knives and guns. Tell me how to use it and how to load and unload the weapons. How to sharpen a knife and how to tell when the knife needs sharpened.

Since time had gone on, I was allowed out and around the crew. I was asked to do small tasks like get beer, clean ashtrays, take out trash, and do random tasks. I got so good at sharpening knifes that I was set at the coffee table with a sharpening stone, a washcloth, and a small cup of water to help keep the stone wet.

As people would stop by, I would check and sharpen their knife for them, yes for the women as well. It was a way to be useful, and a way I could be around others without being picked on or beaten. Another way of protecting myself and be allowed in the house. I would look for validation by going out of my way to do for others so I would be accepted.

This was me taking time out of what I wanted to do for others since I was treated the way I was, just so I could fit in and feel like part of the crew, since I had no one else and no one around wanted me. I just wanted to be accepted and stop the abuse I had to go through.

One day I was outside and one of the friends stopped by with his dog. The man would chain his dog to his truck so no one would see what is inside. He told me the dog was his security for his truck. I did not know what he meant, or why he would need that for his truck, which was was old and dirty. I felt sorry for the dog sitting in the Arizona heat without water. I got a bowl and walked over to the dog. He growled at me and showed his teeth, so I started talking to him. I told him I have water for you and that is all I wanted to give him so please don't bite me. He stopped and backed towards the truck and let me bring water to him. I set the bowl next to him in the shade of the truck so it would not get hot and evaporate. He immediately walked to the water and started drinking. As he finished, he looked at me as if he wanted me to refill the bowl for him, so when I went for the bowl. He walked to me nudging me with his head and allowed me to pet him. I felt the thanks he had for me and we connected. I felt his acceptance of me, and I remember thinking that I finally had a friend and smiled.

For the first time since being in this new place I felt like I was liked. Then as I was petting him and talking to him, two boys on their bikes cut through the parking lot where I was sitting with the dog. It triggered the dog's reaction and he jumped over me to chase the boys for getting too close to the truck. The dog knocked me down, stepped on my body and face, and the chain dragged across my neck, tearing the skin and ripping at my flesh. I screamed, "Stop!" and grabbed the chain. I was dragged for several feet across the parking lot. The boys screamed in fear, and with everything they had within them ran from the dog screaming out they would call the cops and tell their dad.

All I wanted to do was save the boys from the dog getting ahold of them and had I not took the pain and hurt from stopping him, he would have gotten one of the boys. Sitting there bleeding, scratched up and dirty from the seconds of chaos, I was checking to see how bad the damage was. From the noise of everything happening, everyone in the building came out to see what happened. As the man and my mother's boyfriend came running to me, they were screaming at me for getting too close to the truck and dog. I told them what happened, and my mother's boyfriend smacked me down, picked me up and told me to shut up, stop crying and go inside.

The man looked at everyone who was outside and got angry looking at me gritting his teeth and yelling at me for getting to close to his truck. Also, for causing attention and having to leave before the police arrived. I was bleeding, hurt and crying, and all they wanted to do was yell and tell me that is what I get for getting to close to the dog. My neck was scratched up, clothes ripped and dirty, arms and hands scratched, torn, and bleeding.

Alone I had to sit in the bathroom running my hands under water and trying to clean the wounds. I remember thinking of what would have happened to the boy had I not been in the way.

Why had the dog allowed me to sit and pet him, while only his owner was able to?

What was it about me that he felt okay with? Why was I there at that moment to save another?

How was I able to react and know what to do while going through the pain I was going through but still knew to grab the chain and hold on as I did?

These questions ran through my mind while my mother's boyfriend was calling me names and wishing I would 'just disappear one day' so he would be 'rid of me and all my problems'. I knew and felt that no matter what I saved that boy and was strong enough to handle the pain to help others. I looked in the mirror and realized I was a hero and needed no one to tell me otherwise.

Reflection

This would make me feel like I was supposed to go through pain for others so I would feel like a hero and self-validation. If I could take the pain from someone else, then I would feel as if I did something good. It was a way to nurture myself and a way to self sooth after taking on pain.

I would fight others fights, and always look outside of myself to try to help others so I would feel as if I did something right, and no matter what they did to me or what they would say could change this feeling of doing the right thing.

It was a program that I needed so I could validate the pain and survive in new world of darkness. I would rather have love from others even if I had to take or hurt someone else to get the validation.

This young programing will lead to depression, suicidal thoughts, self-worth issues, needing validation, projected anger, self-hate, self-sabotage, and thinking you do not deserve to be happy or deserve love.

You always just want to be loved no matter how bad it is for you. You can end up sacrificing your life by giving your time and energy to others who do not want you to succeed. They will keep you down with them, so they do not feel that you are better than they are.

Taking on others pain and poor choices so you feel like you justified the pain you chose to take on. Making it a habit to think you should always feel this pain because of how you can relate it to love; the only way you learned growing up.

Choose to see what it is you want and or if what is going on has anything to do with you. Others will use you as the root of all their problems, so they never have to admit they are their own.

SEVEN

LEFT TO THE WOLVES

As days went on, I was punished and picked on once again and told how he was going to drop me off in the woods in the mountains and leave me there. "No one wants you, no one cares about you, and all you do is cause problems for your mother." He would tell me how my brother and sister hated me and wanted me out of their life. How he wanted me to get hit by a car, attacked by a drug addict, or fall out of a tree and break my neck.

    I still see his face as he would say these things and wish this into reality. Deep down I could feel the hate and how no one cared about my wounds or how I was being treated. Every day I wanted to run away or try to get back to my father. I asked my mother one time to send me back to my father and I was punished for talking to her like I did by her boyfriend. She tried to tell her boyfriend to stop and she then got smacked and thrown to the couch for yelling at him. I screamed stop and tried to protect her, but without a second thought. I was slapped into the wall and fell to the floor.

    From all the screaming and yelling the police arrived and was asking what happened. All in all, my mother lied to the police and made up a story about how I was acting out and they were sorry for the noise. She let him hit her, beat me. and lied to protect this man. Never did I think she would leave me to the wolves and abandon me like she did in front of me. I thought she was just as scared and did not know what to do after all the abuse I seen her go through.

I could see it in the officer's eyes he knew what was going on and when he asked me if I was okay, I could see her boyfriend look at me with eyes full of hate and the words, *tell them your fine or you will die.*

The way he glared into my soul and gritted his teeth, the muscles in his jaw flexing and bulging from the pressure biting together, the same look he gave me when he would tell me about leaving me in the woods to die, I knew what I had to say; so I said, "Yes sir, I am okay." If I would have told the truth, and he went to jail, he would just find me and kill me anyway after he was released. This man was one of the most violent, ignorant, angry energies I have ever been around. He alone is why I wanted to learn how to be a criminal. Not to steal or take from others, but to one day, when I was big enough, I would murder him in the worst way, and as slow as possible.

When I see myself older and in all black walking the trails, I knew he would use through the woods at night. Catching him off guard knocking him out. Tying him to a tree and cutting his ankles so he could not walk, and letting nature take its course, and letting the animals eat him while he was still alive. I wanted to hear him scream until silence.

Reflection

This was the beginning of all the darkness working its way into my mind and the anger that would fuel, it would add to the darkness. I started to think of all the ways I wanted to kill each of them and made it a game on how I would do it to each person who hurt me or was mean to me.

I was letting the men train me to kill them later in life, and they had no idea what I was thinking, and what I was preparing for. I allowed them to make me a killer and without thinking of how that was so wrong, I was justifying it from what they did to me and my mother.

Thinking of how I could kill him while he slept. Shove a knife in his throat, stab him in the heart, or take his gun and shoot him in the head while he looked at me.

So dark my mind went and so much rage built in my system. I remember the lessons from all the men who would come and go.

How to use a knife. Where to stab. How deep are the organs? How to twist the blade while it is inside the body.

I felt my anger and rage build to the point of liking the thought of killing this man. Smiling at the thought of seeing him in pain and screaming for his life. Finally, I wanted to cause him so much pain and kill him so slow I decided to burn him to death like when he burnt my hand for playing with fire. I wanted to stab him in the legs so he could not move, pour his zippo lighter fluid all over his body and light him up with the same lighter he burned me with.

I was five years old, and he'd successfully created a monster out of me, one who wanted to kill with pleasure, and had no emotions or care of what it would mean for everyone around me.

EIGHT
RAGING FIRE

One day I was looking out back behind our apartment and could see a large tree. I knew the men who would come around would hide in it from the police and the sheriff. I wanted to take something away from them that I knew they loved and made them feel safe.

I never played with lighter fluid before, so I wanted to know how fast it would ignite and how long it would take to kill him. I ran out to the tree, climbed inside, and poured out some liquid on one branch of a pine tree. The flame grew so fast and ran up the branch, I had to dive out of the tree and ran back to the apartment.

I hid on the side of the building and waited to see who would come running first. I heard someone yell out of the back window, and then I ran to the men yelling the pine is on fire. They ran out to see what was happening and they all were yelling, "NO! NO!, NO!" as I sat there watching their faces with anger and disappointment.

I then realized they hid things in there so the police would not find whatever they were hiding, and then realized I took more from them then I knew. The questions then became directed at me. Did you see who did this? Did you go out there and play with fire? Where were you at this whole time? "I was out front where you see me," and then I said, "There was two men who walked by, but I thought they just cut through; and did not see anything until I heard someone yell." Lied I did right to his face, and I see in his eyes he knew it was me.

He told a couple of them to get inside and hide in the bedroom and put something in the air duct. They went in to stash whatever they had and told me to tell the fire department what I had seen and that is all you know. I did what he asked, and after all the chaos later that night, he told me he knows it was me, and he knows because his lighter fluid bottle was missing, and no one else had it.

I told him I was outside; how could I have done it being outside; and I had no way to light it.

He looked at me and said, "I do not need your lies to know you did it, because I see the hate you have in your heart." He said something I will never forget, "You are a bastard child, unwanted and worthless; even your own mother does not want you around. You will be dead or in prison before you are 21 and will never be more than the piece of shit you are right now."

The way he was looking at me hurt me more than the words he said.

For the next month I decided to go all in on my training. Wanted to know all I could so I knew how to beat against any man, or anyone who wanted to hurt me. I asked to be taught how to be a man like them. They laughed and said, "Okay Korey, you think you can handle it, we will show you some things."

I was put through tests and told how to rest; and what to work out when it hurts. How to heal by letting the pain tell your body to work. Drinks lots of water, and how to conceal any weapon I wanted to carry. I was able to help deliver packages of drugs and weapons to other friends, and how to do a 'drop and swap'. Police never look at the kids with back packs. How to breath while running, and how to evade the police if you are being chased. I was also taught the method to hide what you have, so if you get caught, the brothers will know where to look, retracing your path whilst running from the law.

They would teach me how to break into homes and businesses; how to cover my tracks and make it look like I go one way, but really go another. How to wipe down everything and how to load a gun so the bullets do not have my fingerprints on them. How to lose a K-9 unit sent if chased by a dog. Yes, I can evade a dog, and I have done it. They can smell you, but if there is a river or a stream of water, you can jump in and ride it down, or walk in the water as far as you can before you get out on the same side. They always think you cross and never look for you to come back the same way.

The training was so fascinating, and they would always be impressed how fast I would catch on and pick up the skill. I would run obstacles courses and train every day to master my skills and lessons. Martial arts and prison brawl training from an old school Navy Seal. He was a drug addict after he came home from the war and knew my mother and her friends from the time spent on the river living in the woods. He lived in the mountains and refused to be a part of society since he would have flashbacks from his time at war. His focus was clear, and he was always calm. As he would explain the organs and what each one was for, he would speak as if he was telling you how to make pancakes or waffles.

He was the first man I asked how many people he had killed. He left for the night after that and I was beaten good for the disrespect I brought to him. I truly feel okay with that beating for that is not a question you ask a man. That is when I finally realized what I was living for. To kill another man. What am I doing? Why waste my time and energy living to hurt another man who means nothing to me?

Reflection

Thinking like a criminal will never make for a good person. If the person likes the way it feels, the ones who thinks it is fun, and they like it, it is because they were taught this skill and was praised for the work they did. The way Robbin Hood would steal from the rich and give to the poor. Street cats take what they do not have, if they need to survive. Not because they want the image or bragging rights. We only take what we need.

When a criminal takes for pleasure, and because they want to take from others, it is because they have a hatred for the ones that do have. They were taught that these people do not deserve these things they take for granted, and that they are bad people who deserve it.

This is a template that needs to be exposed and talked about. Understand, if for generations people believe they are stuck in the life they are born into, they will never try to be more than what they were told.

The only way I was shown love, or acceptance, in this life was for me to go out and take from others. If you cannot relate, or understand, and you judge because you never had to feel this way, I understand; but how would they be able to see through your eyes when you are not able to see through the eyes of a street cat?

Just remember the training, and the things you have been taught, are the judgments you place on others. The way the training works for anyone at this age, is the feelings they would feel during love or hate.

If when they did something bad, they would be praised and loved they will only know how to replicate the feeling by doing the action. If you are always praised to be a criminal, you will like the feelings of being called one. All the training, and all the things I did was to fit in and survive as best I could.

These were all old habits and blockages that ruled all my life, until I changed into who I really am, after I was able to see with my own eyes, not with what they taught me.

NINE
3RD EYE OPEN

One day, my sister wanted to get something out of the cabinet and told me to help her get what she wanted. I asked what it was, she told me it was gum, and I wanted a piece as well. So, I helped her by letting her stand on my back, get on the counter so she could stand up and open the door. We were home alone that day so no one would see, and we had to hurry before anyone came back.

She opened the cabinet, got a piece of gum, and teased me by enjoying it and making sounds as she chewed on it, waving my piece back and forth. I yelled to give me one and she finally dropped one. I went for the gum, and the lower cabinet door was open from us using it as a step. As I went down, I hit my head right between my eyes splitting my head open. The corner of the cabinet door opened my skull right between my eyes. I put my hand over the hole. As I looked down at my hand, I saw blood fill the palm of my hand and screamed.

My sister jumped down and I ran to the bathroom to look at it. My face was covered with blood running down my face. I could see into my head as the hole opened and closed. I was crying and thinking I could die. There was blood all over the floor and I started to fade. Everything got blurry as well as the blood getting into my eyes. I sat down on the toilet and leaned back as my sister and brother called 911.

I do not remember much, except for seeing a lot of people and was rushed to the hospital. Faded memories of people being nice to me and calling me such a strong little man and how I was doing so good. I loved this place where they treated you so nice, and say hi and hello every time they would see me. Even if I know I haven't seen them before they were so nice and loving. It was short lived, and I had to leave with my mother after I was patched up and stitched. There was no joy I can remember on that ride home.

There was a lot of questions asking why I did what I did, and why do I always have to cause problems.

My sister told everyone I made her get up there, and said I was crying and screaming for her to get me the gum I was told I was not allowed to have. It was my mothers and I was not to have what was hers. I was not allowed to talk back and explain that I did not do anything but ask to have a piece like she did. All I wanted was a piece of gum, and that I did not like her teasing me with it.

She was so mad at me, and when I got back to the apartment everyone there was making fun of my bandages and asking if the poor little baby was okay? Laughing at the teddy bear one of the nurses gave me so I would feel better. They were saying, "Do not fall on your way to the room and get the police called again; and stop acting like you're hurt. Suck it up and I bet you will learn your lesson about climbing on the counter."

Only me and my sister knew what happened, and she told them I climbed up and fell off the counter onto the cabinet. She lied so she would not be in trouble. No one would listen or wanted to hear me speak. I was still in pain, so I went to my room where my brother was and stayed to myself. My brother was a reader and did not talk to me much, and so I was able to stay to myself and try to heal in peace.

Each day was one of teasing and messing with me while I was trying to heal. My head was hurting so much. To move around caused me pain and all I wanted to do was sleep. I remember having bad dreams and waking up scared and crying.

Seeing my mother's face covered in blood and memories of the kitchen floor covered in blood with red handprints on the wall and the phone. I would see people standing in my room when no one was there and at night I would hear voices talking into my ear. Whispers in the darkness and sometimes I would hear the gunshot, like the one on the way to Arizona from the man we picked up.

Other nights I would close my eyes and see a bright light as if someone were shining a flashlight in my face, but when I would open my eyes, no one was there. When I would ask about it, or try to tell anyone about it, they would tell me to shut up and go away, hearing nothing I would say.

While still healing I was also in trouble for bringing the police and child protective services. I was already disliked so much for something I had no idea of. I was always told it was my fault and that I was such a bad child. All I wanted was to know why I was so different.

One night while trying to sleep one of the men walked in the room all of us kids where in and pulled out his penis and peed on the wall behind the door as if he were in the bathroom. When I told him to stop the man replied to shut up and asked me why I was in there. My brother told him he was in our room and when he realized what he was doing he just started laughing and finished anyway then walked out.

The next morning, I told my mother what had happened, and the room smelled like pee for the rest of the four months we had to live there. The wall was yellow and the carpet stained, we had to live like that until we finally were evicted for all the noise complaints and all of the problems we have caused.

It was shortly after that we had to find another place to live. The daily practice was for me to stay out of the way, and if my mother's boyfriend or friends saw me, I would have to do pushups, sit ups, or hold the prone position until my arms would give out.

At only five years old, they would push me around, smack me in the head, and sometimes if they were drunk enough, they would make me stand still chest out and they would give me six to eight inch punches to the chest to toughen me up. "Get up stop crying and if you do not stop crying, we will hit you more and much harder. Boys do not cry, boys do not feel, boys take what they want and will kill anyone who challenges them."

They would tell me how I will be raped and murdered when I go to prison. Stories of the kids who go missing and what condition the bodies are found in later in the woods. They showed me what to do if someone snatches me and tries to put me in a van or car. They showed me where to shove the knife, and how to twist it so the hole will not close, and how to always have a way out of any situation. No matter how big or strong someone is, they all have a weakness and in such a scenario how to keep breathing and keep calm enough to find a way to get out of it; or take them with you if you must die. Never will I be killed without taking at least one with me on my way out.

I was a trained killer thief fueled by anger and rage against the world who rejected me. If I was to not have friends, then I would be feared so no one would hurt me again. This mindset pattern would stay with me into my thirties and with all friends and family.

So much pain and hate this man had for me, and my own mother chose to keep this kind of male role model around for me to be raised by. So many times, I wanted to kill him or to kill myself. I remember thinking about walking into the woods at night and keep going until something killed me or walking off the edge of a cliff. So many times, I remember wanting to leave but had nowhere to go or any friends to run to. I was alone and did not want to be there anymore.

The whole time I was going through each of these trials and lessons I was not able to see or understand why they hated me, or why I was the one treated so different for things I did not know I did. I was never asked how I was doing, or if I wanted to go do anything.

One of the only games I can think of that these men would play with me is a game called trust. A game where you stand still, and they throw a knife in the ground next to your foot. If you do not move or jump, you get to throw back. I learned quickly to accept my fate and stand still because I watched these men throw knifes and they always hit the right spot. Hours and hours a day throwing knifes and practice flipping them. I learned not to flinch and got to throw back. They would stand there and say, "Go ahead."

These men would give me a chance to stab them accepting and fully understanding what they were allowing me to do. I knew if I hit them, all they would do is stab me back to teach me to hit my target or there would be consequences. I never tried to hit them, throwing the knife out far enough. They knew I was not going to try to hit them or stab them with the knife.

Reflection

Not thinking I mattered, I would go through life thinking I was not worth saving and that began the programming that if I did not take care of myself, I would not survive. Always believing no one cared and no one wanted me around. I was programming that if I did not do for others, they would cast me out. I would believe if someone were being nice to me, it was because they wanted something from me, or for me to do something for them.

I did not have any friendships, so I did not know how to have social skills. Leading to me telling others about my truth and opinion without thinking what it would make others feel like. No consideration for other people's feelings or emotions, as well as never caring about anything that happened to others.

If you find yourself not caring for others and hate being around people, look back and feel into how you were brought up?

A lot of friends and family loving you and treating you with love and acceptance, Or was it closer to mine?

During childhood we can be programmed into being emotionless physical bodies that react only to low vibes and feeds off the weakness of others. It is a learned condition, not how you are. This is not really you. In your natural state as a baby, you feel love and smile when someone is happy to see you.

While the body is growing, it is being programmed with the emotional energy in the home. What attaches most to a child is the state of the energy surrounding them during these years of development. Mine was one of hate and fear with the instinct to survive. Always on alert and ready for the worst thing to happen. This will not help you enjoy life or be able to pay attention to the beauty of what this life must see and experience.

To look back now and see that all the things those men did to me, I now know this all happened for a reason. To look at this small amount of time in my life, I can see all of what it has done to me later in life.

How for so many years, the level of anger and dark thoughts I would think, was from this time. I was conditioned to hate and think all the negative thoughts I was thinking. Now I see how it was taught and the energy I was surrounded by.

When I would see this is what life was like, it was as if I agreed to this, and this is how I must be also. I did not realize that they must have had something similar, or maybe worse happen to them.

I do not know and do not care anymore. I now appreciate knowing I can choose to be nothing like them, and to choose to love others while they are on their own journey.

We always form opinions about others and even if you know just enough of the story to make a judgment, we never really take the time to look deeper, or ask the questions that make people uncomfortable. I know what happened to me in this beginning stage was to wake me up to reality, and to not see the world through a false filter, making me believe it is as easy or that bad things don't happen to people or children.

I was shocked, and awakened, to a world of people that think they live in a reality, when now I see they were taught they are supposed to be this way, with no one ever showing them differently.

So, I invite you to look deeper when you judge someone else for their opinions or the choices they make. You never know what all someone else has been through, whether they'll tell you the whole truth, or you just have an opinion about someone else's way of life.

This is not the last I would face, but I have healed and forgiven him and the men for believing what they did was to be okay. I know they hated themselves, and that is why they did what they did. They all have their own demons to deal with; and I will not allow this way of teaching and training to be passed down to the next.

I am not them.

This is not saying any of this is okay, but I am saying when I go back and can see what I went through, I know why. There is something in each lesson for all of us to learn in every situation.

The trick is to try to find a way to see the reason it is happening, and to look at it without feeling the pain and suffering. Ask yourself deep down, if you were to know the reason this happened to you, what would it be?

If you are in a space of open honest curiosity, the answer will reveal itself to you, and you will feel the understanding of the universal law. Cause and effect, yin, and yang.

The reasons are of your own; and if you find yourself judging your choices from the past decision, or something you did, I ask you to see the lesson in the choice, or experience, without judgment or opinion, and look to know the reason why.

You may know right away, or you may need to investigate it and dig deep. Take the time needed to see what you need to see and feel what you need to feel.

Once you can do that, you will be able to request to your subconscious mind to let that memory attached to pain and blockages go, and to detach from any of its negative energy. You are in control of what holds you back, and you can manifest your reality. The question is, are ready to call it to the surface and release yourself from the pain?

I believe in you and know you can so if you need to, borrow some of my faith in you. Know you are capable of anything you want to achieve; and that you are enough as you are, to have whatever you want in this life.

Our natural state is of bliss and if you are not happy with what has happened to you, or there is a memory you feel is holding you back, confront it and pull it to the surface. Know this will not define you or your choices. You are in control; and if you need time to dig it up and find out why this keeps coming up for you then do it. Take the time and find yourself. Make time for you to just be you. Make time to see what it is that you want and how you want to feel. Simply ask yourself, "Am I happy with my current situation?" Also ask, "What is it that is holding me back?"

If there are subjects you do not like to think about or talk about, find space and time to really investigate why. These are the first signs that you need to deal with it, and anything that is scary, or brings fear, is a blockage that you want to remove.

Always know that if something is scary then it is something working to hold you back, and you can choose to remove it by facing it.

Do not ever think anything that happens to you, or any experience you have been through in your life, is one that can hold you back. Yes, things are hard and sometimes difficult to deal with or understand. If you look at these situations as happening ***for you*** instead of to you, then you will be able to see it differently.

Some blockages can take more time. When working through layers, always remember to take your time and to never rush a healing process.

If you make the effort, and keep working towards what you genuinely want, and know you are capable of achieving, then you will not fail. You will see, feel, and know you are whatever you truly desire to be.

My past in this beginning stage holds a lot of the energy I carried throughout my life and I can now see what the lessons for me were. I held the belief I was worth nothing and deserved the pain I went through. This was my filter of life.

When we put our energy and mindset that we are only what others portray us as, or tell us what we are, then we will be what someone else decided.

Others will project onto you what they want to you to see yourself as, not realizing it is they who do not want you to ever be better than they are, and they will try to hold you back.

This happens on a subconscious level, and others do not always know what they are doing. They have their own filters and blockages that they must live with and work through. Really look at the person who *you feel* is making you feel less, then try to see if they are just hiding from how they feel on the inside.

Do not let others make you feel any other way. If you do not like what someone else makes you feel like, and if they are just trying to be mean, let them deal with their own issues and know you are enough. If what makes you happy does not hurt others, or stops others from living their life, then you are living your life as you want, and no one should make you feel bad about it.

Learn to control your own mind and emotions and if they get triggered, look into why? If you doubt or judge yourself look deep down inside into why you feel this way. Is this what you think? Or, is this something someone else has projected? Do not take on what others want you to be. Just be you.

TEN

THE INITIATION

This new place we moved into became a haven for so many criminals, and for anyone who wanted a place to crash. My mother would tell people she was Momma Cat and would take care of all these people.

While working she would also go to food shelters and get free boxes of food and bring back for us to eat and got food stamps as well. So many people coming and going, other people who had kids would come over and stay with us.

Still five years old, some of my sister's friends would stay the night and while others were sleeping, they would sneak over and get in bed with me on the floor. They would start touching my stomach and then slide their hands down my pants pulling them down, playing with my penis. They would get it hard and put it in their mouth then climb on top of me putting it inside of them. Telling me to just relax and that I will like it. Talking me through the whole experience. I like girls and I did like the attention. I did not think it was wrong because I was never told that it was. Once my sister found out what they were doing, she made me sleep in the room with her so she could see what they were doing. These sisters from the trailer park took advantage of me, and even my own sister wanted to learn. I was the testing subject and did not really know what was happening but since I liked my sister's friends, I thought that this was something people did.

I was being used for sexual taboo with two sisters as well as my own. They would teach each other how to give oral sex using me each night they stayed over. My sister would sometimes make me sleep in her room so she could do the same when we were alone. Everyone had no idea; except the girls my sister would bring over to use me. All I wanted was to be accepted and not picked on.

This happened a lot in the place we lived in, from all the stories I would hear; and sometimes I would witness firsthand. Some evenings when the adults would leave us home alone and go to the bar, we would run around the neighborhood sneaking around and looking to see what was going on. I would see people walking around naked in their yard. Men and women having sex in some of the weirdest places.

Also, there were other kids around the park doing the same thing. Learning this from what we saw in and out of the home, these were our day to day lessons, and we were not being told if it was wrong or if it was bad. If anything, when we would get caught as kids playing with each other, the adults would laugh and say things like "at least he is not gay" and "she has to learn sometime". In a way they would support the notion that this is okay, or just what happened instead of talking about it and explaining.

I would spend most of the time with the wizards and witches of the park, and the warlocks who would teach me about crystals and natural energy. We would hear stories of witches in the woods behind us in the hills, and the tales of children never coming out of the woods again.

I would try to go out into the woods late at night when everyone else would be asleep, or out for the night. I could see fires on top of the hill late at night and hear singing, and was captivated by this sound and was drawn in. I remember hearing womens screams and howls in the nights of a full moon and others telling us to stay inside. When we would ask "why" or "what are they doing out there?", we would be told to stay away from the crazy people in the woods, and to never ask for help from a stranger in the woods if we ever run into anyone out there. Just say, "No thank you and be nice, walk away and do not look them in the eyes." Such childrens tales and stories we all thought.

Days after that, I started seeing people walking in the woods behind us. I would be outside and see them as they would be walking through the woods and they would stop and look at me. As if they could tell I was watching them. I had the strangest feelings, but I was not scared, simply curious to what and who they were.

One of the men I will never forget was a man everyone called Evil. He had long blond hair, always wore all black and had a light brown trench coat. His eyes were bright blue, and he had fangs like a vampire. I will never forget the way he could look deep into your soul and when he smiled at you, it was a hypnotizing feeling that you could not look away. Everyone else was afraid of him and did not like when he was around. I would watch him all the time and was always around when he was over. I liked how I could see people, as well as grown men, be afraid of him and not want to sit by him or talk to him. He would catch me watching him, and he would just smile back and go on about what he was doing.

One night he was curious and asked me what it was I wanted to know? I would always watch him, and he could see my interest. Other kids were afraid of him, but I wanted to be more like him. I liked how he would scare others and I wanted to do the same so I would stop being picked on and beaten all the time.

Once I told him this, he laughed and asked me if I was sure I wanted to know what it was like to be what he was? I said yes, I do not want anyone to be able to hurt me anymore. He took me outside and walked me to the fire pit in the yard and told me to sit have a seat. He told me that he was a vampire, but not like in the stories or the silly tales people tell. He told me he was over 600 years old, and he knew what I was. When I asked him what he meant by that, he simply smiled and said, "One day you will know. I cannot tell you; you must find it on your own, and you must allow it to come to you." He told me that I have special blood and he could smell it. He made a fire and told me to stare into the fire and do not look away no matter what. As I did, the man started to speak in gibberish or a language I did not understand. I could see him moving around both the fire and me while speaking in this language. I did not see anything in the fire but after a couple of minutes he stood behind me, placed his head on the back of my head and started to growl like a lion.

A cold chill ran through my whole body and I felt lightheaded as if I were going to pass out. The low vibration made me start to shake a little and I started to get scared. Then he told me to close my eyes. As I did, I could see the fire in my mind dancing like I was seeing it in real time. He then roared like a lion, and the energy that flooded every cell of my body was like being on fire. The man bit me on the back part of my neck and grabbed me by the throat. Shaking me back and forth, but I did not open my eyes. It did not hurt at all. I was so shocked and scared, and to describe the feeling that came over me, it would be like a rollercoaster. He let me go and I fell to the ground next to the fire and felt like I was completely drained and could pass out asleep on the ground in the dirt next to the fire. I tried to look up, and he was leaning back looking to the stars and growling. I remember him helping me up and taking me back inside, where I slept for the rest of the night.

I never saw him again and no one ever heard from him. Strange things started happening during the evenings after that, and I would have the strangest dreams. I would see greyish men carrying my body out of the room and taking me to a bright place. By the next morning I would wake up in different places in the house and would ask if anyone carried me or if I was sleepwalking? They would tell me no and look at me like I was crazy. One time I was told I woke up, sat up, and was looking around the room. They asked me what was wrong and told me I was pale white, and my eyes looked black. They said I scared them just by looking this way and seemed as if I was not there. I then fell back and went back to sleep as if nothing happened.

Other times I woke up outside on the front porch sitting in a chair. One night I walked into my brothers' room to get some sleep while the adults were partying in the living room. I saw a face in the window looking at me. I ran into the living room telling everyone someone was looking in. They grabbed weapons and they ran around outside looking to see who it was. No one was there and no footprints to see. They asked if I was seeing things or if I was lying. I told them, "No," and showed them were I seen it, and on the glass was a couple smudges from where it looked like someone leaned against the window. There were no footprints but there was evidence of something touching the window. I never went into that room again.

At night you could hear footsteps walking on the roof and through the trailer as if someone were there, even though it was just us kids while the adults were out. This was just another thing to add to the list of things going on at the trailer we lived in. Once we started to ask the other kids in the park about this, they told us that a man was killed in the trailer we lived in, and that no one wanted to live there because of it. That is why my mother got a good deal on the rent.

This was a place that held dark energy and I started to notice it more and more. I started talking to people about the tales and the stories of the Skinwalkers (In Navajo culture, a skin-walker (Navajo: yee naaldlooshii) is a type of harmful witch who has the ability to turn into, possess, or disguise themselves as an animal. The term is never used for healers.) and the sightings near the reservations or out in the desert. How the shapeshifters (is the ability to physically transform through an inherently superhuman ability, divine intervention, demonic manipulation, sorcery, spells or having inherited the ability) were everywhere, and to speak their name, would invite them to see you, and be called to taunt you or your family. There are stories of how ranchers would shoot a coyote, or a wolf, and when they went to see if it were dead, the animal would stand up like a man and run off. Other stories of the shapeshifters would run at the rancher after being shot and the rancher would shoot it again killing the man. Then once the rancher would go look, it would be just a coyote dead shot several times, and the rancher would tell about how it stood like a man and ran at him. This place was like the twilight zone for people who did not live here, but these stories we would hear, were just part of life.

ELEVEN

THE HUNTERS MOON

We bounced around from place to place and had to put our things in storage. We only had what we could pack in a trash bag and carry to and from anywhere. We would stay with my mother's friends, and sometimes, people related to the family did not want me around.

I loved the cowboys and ranchers we would stay with, since they had a lot of animals. My mother's boyfriend was not allowed to stay at certain places with us, as he was known and was not liked in town.

I would work with the animals and try to help the ranches as much as I could. They would tell me how good of a worker and helper I was. This made me want to help even more and learn more. I would wake up early and be outside with the cattle men and the boys who would line up the animals and feed them. I would watch and study what they would do and how they would handle themselves while working with the animals and horses. I would talk to the animals and loved helping clean them and take care of the stalls. I did not mind the work because they always seemed to like having me around. When we stayed at other homes, I would help take out the trash and clean up the house and again I was complimented and sometimes treated with ice cream or a cup cake.

I would find any way I could to get the positive reaction from anyone new, and if I wanted something, I would offer to work for what I wanted.

Everyone in and around town knew what my mother had me out of wedlock and most of the town was related to the family she married into. A lot of people did not like that I was the bastard child of my mother, and the disrespect I brought to their family, but they did see that I was a helper, and all I wanted was to be allowed to be around them without being beaten or punished.

At night I would sneak out and watch the stars and moon as it would change its course and shape. I felt at ease and connected to the light as if I were able to leave this place and go somewhere else for a short time. One of the full moons that was out while staying with a rancher, the man seen me outside at night alone looking up. He came out to me and asked, "What did you see?"

I told him I like the moon, and when I can see it as if it was day, from the amount of light the full moon showered down, I felt happy. The man told me it was called a Hunter's Moon. It was the first full moon after the Harvest Moon. I was so fascinated about the different phases of the moon and the names he would tell me. He showed me star clusters, and told me about the Milky Way, and how the planets move around the sun, and the moon around the earth.

This was the first time anyone was teaching me something different for the lessons I had been learning, and the training I was going through with the other men in my life. I have so much love and respect for the cowboys and ranchers I was able to meet, giving me a little hope that all men and people in my life are not the same. I was hopeful there might be a way I can have a better life if I was able to live with any of them. They loved their children, and would have time together, teaching and helping and giving. Watching all these different families and home life events I was able to see, made me feel so lucky to have them in my life. Then, since my mother wanted to get back to her boyfriend, we had to leave. She was able to get a place, so we had to move into this new place which I had no idea was going to be one of the darkest times in my life.

All my mother wanted was this man who beat me and treated her like a dog. She would say, "I want to live my life my way and with who I want. No one will tell me different. I do not care what anyone thinks or has to say about my choices." She never involved us kids or cared what I was living through. It was all about what she wanted, and right when I was getting hopeful that I might have a chance at a better life, it was changed again.

Time to adapt or die was the saying around the people that my mother decided to be around and live with. This new place that she moved us into was behind a strip mall that had a store, a church, and a furniture shop. Across the street was a library, and thrift shop next to it. At least this place had things for me to go see. Behind the two-story building, that was two apartments, there was a large open field that had horses. I was able to go get grass and feed horses and watch them run back and forth through the field.

There was a house next to us and my mother knew the neighbors. I liked going over there for the wild berries that would grow along the fence. They had kids I could be friends with They always had a lot of people over and they would bring their kids, so I was able to meet new people. I had better hope and was looking forward to meeting new people and making new friends, like I thought I would make when we jumped from house to house. I did not know that I would be so wrong, and how my life was going to change.

It was a place I refined my training while listening and watching others, learning to live in the dark. I remember opening a box of cereal and pouring out roaches into my bowl. At night when I would go to use the bathroom and turn on the light, you could see them scatter and run up the walls. If you left a drink out for too long or overnight, it would be filled with dead roaches floating in the cup by morning. This was acceptable to my mother, and the people she chose to be around. The extent of not caring, the amount of pain that would be inflicted on me every day while trying to survive, was also acceptable.

When I was at the age of going to school, I wanted to get out of the situation so bad; but during this time the gang wars began, and it was a time of fight or die in the street of Arizona. Gangster life and thug life where raging. Drugs and guns were as much currency as honor and loyalty. I was trained in how much bags weigh and what product is what and how to roll joints for my older brothers and sisters. In the streets you are taught, blood relatives mean nothing to the family you develop during the worst times in your life. The trials and lessons create a bond only true street cats understand. We would watch others steal and take from other families, justifying the act by segregation and hate for the working class. Adults would have sex in front of us kids, drunk and with no care. Older girls using me for practice, looking and playing with what I had. I learned foreplay and was having sex at six years old, as if it were normal. How quick everything was working and ready. The energy put into having sex and surviving was daily and a way out of the reality of the current situation, and a way to feel good, as the way it feels while in union or play. Parents and older kin would do it anywhere and everywhere. Outside, in the kitchen, living room, and you could hear them in the bedroom if they made it there. We knew to stay quiet or act like we were asleep for we would be punished if we got up or told them to stop. I did not have my own room, and mostly slept in the living room in the corner; or was always put away from everyone to figure it out as we moved around.

Some of my sister's friends would play 'house' and would undress me and do all of the things to me. I, being a boy, liked girls and loved the attention. After that, I would play all I could and use this time to feel as if I were finally wanted, or a feeling of being loved. I was a cute boy, and a lot of girls liked me.

The older boys would treat me like a little brother and use me to crawl in windows, get into doggy doors and unlock the house we would break into and steal from. I finally felt I had a purpose and a family was growing around me. To get positive attention I would steal from others and give to my street family. This was why I got so good at stealing and taking from others. I started to up the work and look at stealing more and more. This was the time I decided to take the world so everyone would want me around. Kicking in doors of stores and other gift shops, as well as other's homes. We would watch others in the area, and we could tell what time and how long families would be gone. We knew what to look at, where to stash what we stole, and how long to wait before we went to sell it just in case the police came looking. Everyone knew who the bad kids were, but we also knew how to hide it; and try to get away with it.

Some lessons where harder than others.

School made life difficult, and even there I would steal food and crafts, as well as others school supplies because other kids had nice things. I wanted nice things and my mother would not get it for me, so I would take it from others. I never asked for much. She would get angry with me if I did ask and tell me I do not need it or, "No, I am not getting you that." I rarely took showers, and never had more than one pair of pants and two shirts. Socks where a luxury, and shoes that fit where a blessing.

My mother would go to churches and food drives to get free things for us kids and lie to churches about how many kids she had so they would give more food. She would use fake IDs and hit multiple shelters to take all she could get. Her theory was 'Why work for it if you can get it for free? Make people feel sorry for you and they will give you something'. Even when they had to shave my head for having lice, we would go to Pizza Hut and people would give us food. Later finding out she told them I had cancer and we did not have the money to eat. I see it as survival, and others will see her as evil. While in this place I learned to become a master thief and robber. I was taught to look at someone's shoes or watch to tell if they had money, and how to follow people without them knowing they are being watched and followed. I was taught how to make others feel bad about your life, ask them for money, or help to take from others. I was taught to go to the grocery store and ask for a quarter so I could call for a ride home. If you got 20 people to do that within a few hours, I would have the money to eat food off the dollar menu. If that were not working, I learned to steal food from the store, and how to eat food in the store where no one would see, and then leave. I never wasted much time on candy. I liked real food and not just snacks. Plus, the candy was up front, and people would watch me up there. I would put items in my waistline and hold in my stomach and fill all I could in the area between my shirt and stomach. If I were ever caught, I could outrun anyone who tried to catch me, and would always evade any opponent. Even the police could not catch me. I knew the woods and paths better than most and could see in the dark better than anyone around me.

When you are raised in a home or trailer with no electricity, or live in the woods, your eyes adapt, and you evolve as you need to survive. Many times, I could stand still in the dark and police and people would walk right past and never see me, as I watch them look for me. I loved when they would look right at me and I could see their eyes and see them look at me, but not be able to see me back at all. I was becoming what they were training me to be without knowing any other life was possible. I was a master at anything I put my mind to, and I had no distractions like video games or friends to waste time from my survival.

Times were always dark, and I was always on alert and ready for anything. When every day you never know what is going to happen, or how you are going to eat, each day becomes a survival of the fittest, and ready to take from others. If you were in the way of one of the men my mother kept around, you could fall prey to anything. They would take my bounty and never share with me. If I stole food from a delivery truck and brought it back, I would get last pick of what was inside. I would wait until the delivery driver would load his cart and roll the load inside, counting how long it would take for him to return. As he would go into the store I would start counting as I jumped into the truck and grabbed anything I could and then run with it. I had one truck a week I knew I could take from, and what the delivery days of the week were. I would steal from anyone that left me the opportunity, but I never stole if I did not have to. I did not like doing it, but I knew I had to if I was to survive. Until it was all I knew and would start to take from the ones around me, to stop them taking from me.

I remember wanting to know why I was always differently treated and told to leave or go away, and my brother and sister never got treated as such. I was the one everyone could hate and there was nothing I could do about it. I remember how they would tell me how bad of a kid I was, and that I was the reason for their problems. My own mother would say if it were not for you, I would be fine, and everyone would not hate me. I should have left you with your dad. I asked her to send me away and told her to do it, but she said she could not. Confused and alone I did not understand why I was such a problem, and why they would not let me leave. I would try to find ways to run away but had no idea where to go and if I were caught, I would be brought back to them and punished for bringing the police around.

Reflection

I chose to see my mother as a lost soul, hating herself enough to not care how she gets by. In these times, she had no self-confidence and no positive people truly making her see what she was doing wrong. Most people would give and just tell her what she was doing instead of making her work for it and cut off her handouts. She was conditioned to ask, instead of forced to work extra and stop the drugs.

One thing food stamp's do not buy is alcohol and drugs. She worked for her fix, not for her kids. This is not to make excuses, but to make sure you know she knows she is wrong, and that will not change.

What I ask is to understand this was taught to her, and without the right guidance she will teach this to others as she has in her life and so on.

This time in my life would solidify the programming of a criminal, and the dark times I would hold inside, I would start to believe I was what they were teaching me to be; and what I was supposed to become in their eyes.

The pain forms the hate, it would make me a monster towards others, and I would have no remorse for the actions I would take stealing. I would only love and be loved by other children that lived were I did and would live their story and lives from the tales and nightmares we all lived through on a day to day basis. It would set a default system of self-destructive patterns and would confirm to the child from the teachings and lessons we were to receive. Though I knew it was not right, what choice do you have at five/six years old.

To get along you must go along. To survive you must be part of the pack or be cast out with no way of surviving. Living in a situation where all the kids around you are talking about suicide and how they tried to do it, or thought about it, will paint a dark picture of life. This is what we all thought was a reality, and a way of life like everyone else had to make it through.

The blockage is in the details of the conditioning and energy surrounding you. If you are taught a habit, then it is not your habit. You only choose to continue if you do not see any other way or opportunity.

TWELVE
BIRTHDAY REALITY

On my seventh birthday I was playing outside, and some new friends came over to see my mother and her boyfriend. I was so happy it was my birthday because I thought I would get something for it, like the other kids always did. I told this new couple it was my birthday and they asked, "What did you get?"

I said, "Nothing yet," and they looked at my mother and she glared back at me.

I did not know I had hurt her feelings for saying that, and she said, "You will get it later."

I stayed outside like I was supposed to during the day for only adults are allowed in the house during the day. Later when I asked her if I can have my gift, she said, "I did not get you anything. I cannot afford it."

So, I walked away and one of her friends said, "Here you go Korey," and handed me a five-dollar bill.

I was so shocked and said, "Thank you so much," and felt like the richest kid in the world! I got to not only go to the store, but buy whatever I wanted to get for myself, not knowing five dollars value. I put it in my back pocket and went back outside until it was time for bed and fell asleep. The next morning, I woke up and went to get the five dollars out of my back pocket and it was gone. I looked and looked and could not find it. I was so upset that I lost it somehow while I was sleeping. I asked if anyone had seen it and everyone said no. I felt so bad I lost the gift from that lady and now I get nothing for my birthday. I noticed some beer bottles in the kitchen and knew they did not have any money, so I asked where did those come from?

My sister said, "They went out to get them last night after you fell asleep. Mom had a five-dollar bill, so she walked to the store and got them." She told me, "Mom took it out of your pocket while you were asleep and said you do not need it."

I still can feel the pain I felt in my chest and the dark shadow that followed knowing my mother stole from me to get her and her boyfriend beer on my birthday with a gift from a stranger. I wanted to die, and that was the first time I tried to kill myself at six years old. I walked out to a tree and used the dog chain that was our neighbors and climbed the tree and tied it to a high branch. I wanted this tree so when they walked outside, they could see I would no longer be a burden on this family. I wanted to display my dead body hanging from the tree so they would see me as they walked out of the apartment. No more abuse or pain. No more being in the way. No more problem child to complain about.

As I wrapped the chain around me, so I could climb up above the branch I was standing on to get it around my neck, I slipped off the branch and fell out of the tree. I fell sideways, and while the chain locked around my stomach, I could barely breathe and tried to scream, but the chain squeezed the air out of me. Just before I was about to black out, one of the neighbor's friend's saw what happened and ran to me, lifted me up and undid the chain.

Catching my breath and crying he asked, "What were you doing?"

I told him I slipped and fell while trying to hang myself because I did not want to live anymore. His face was in shock and he was getting angry and gritted his teeth, looking at the apartment I was living in, knowing all who were inside. As people came out because of the noise of him yelling for help and me crying, he told them he had got me. When I was asked what happened the neighbor's friend said I was trying to make a swing and slipped.

He lied for me, told me I would be okay, to go sit in the shade and calm down telling me, "Do not ever try that again." He took the chain with him so I could not.

Everyone told me I was stupid and that is what I get. Laughing and saying, "dumb ass kid" and "that boy is stupid". I sat there for hours with no one who cared about the pain I was in and how they took the first money I was ever given to buy beer for themselves. I can still see and hear the trees I would stare at thinking of another way I could get away or try to kill myself again.

Reflection

This was a blockage of anger and rage powered by pure pain, and since I was not able to cry or have a way to release this memory, I would have to hold it down deep and sit with the fact I was bad at trying to even kill myself. It was as if God wanted me to be here and go through all this pain.

I put judgement and hate for others who would go to church and seemed to have a great life, yet I was forced to live in this one. My blockage was built on the priceable fact I was not able to get out of the situation, or away from these evil low vibe men and women, who I had no idea had to live life possibly harder, and with more pain than I did.

I did not take the time to listen to the stories of how bad it was for them, and what all they had to go through. I was so deep in only how I felt, and what I was going through and did not care what it was they would talk about. The beatings and raping's the adults who raised us had went through during their youth. What all they went through when they were young. The shacks and tents they had to live in. The poor poverty hate that was taught by the angry men who had to work and do whatever he could to provide. Numbing the pain with alcohol and drugs they were led off the path and taught the same teaching they are carrying on.

They do not know the difference and cannot see without someone caring enough for them to show them. Even today, I see parents teaching kids what they learned when they were young, not realizing times have changed and you should make new rules and new standards for the youth to develop in. If you want your child to exceed you and have more than you did at their age, you should probably encourage them to seek their own truth. If you are not happy with your childhood, then why do you teach it to your children?

Ergo the reflection.

THIRTEEN
THEY ARE REAL IF YOU ARE OPEN TO IT

Something was wrong and I felt something was different. I never fell out of trees. I was a great climber. I have climbed that tree so many times and never fell out. I stated to play what happened over and over and then realized I felt pushed. Like a wind shoved me while I was wrapping the chain around me so I could climb up one more branch and jump. I felt it through my entire body and felt something did not let me do it. I felt I was supposed to be saved and needed to know why. Every time I would think about it, I felt afraid and cold chills ran down my back. I could not figure it out. I just wanted to go away and not be around the people I was forced to be with.

    Night after night I would sit alone for hours and stare at the moon and night sky, watching the stars. Some girls from the neighborhood would sit with me and we would talk about all kinds of things. We would question what all it is about and if there was more out there in the stars, or if the stories where true about the creatures in the mountains people would talk about. We would watch the sky for hours, and a lot of the time the girls would end up using me for sexual games and play.

    Things became the norm and we all had our differences and opinions about it, but it was learning nonetheless. We saw what our parents did and how they acted, and we did what we felt like doing. The girls around me loved me for some reason, and would talk to me about all kinds of feelings and things that would happen to them, and the older men who would do sexual things to them; or what they would make the girls do to them. I was a place for them to run to if they needed to cry and release, I was someone they could love, or feel as if they could tell anything to me. My family became those who wanted me around, and the reason I felt I was saved from the tree. I started to feel my purpose was to be there for others who needed me, and I wanted to feel wanted, so I started looking outwards for the attention. I wanted to feel love and acceptance.

Night after night I would hear my mother fighting and yelling and sometimes, she would scream and yell. I hated my life and feeling like there was nothing I could do. I would look to what I could do to help, but I knew he would kill me if I tried to do anything to save her. All I was wanting was for us to drive back to my father so all this pain would stop. One night they were fighting, and my mother tried to leave. As she got some things together and tried to head to the door, her boyfriend picked up a frying pan from the kitchen and threw it at her head. She moved and the pan hit the front door bounced off the door and knocked me out. All I can remember was that I could not walk, and everything was blurry, but I do know the police showed up and took him away. My head hurt for the whole next day and I felt sick when I opened my eyes. The next day I was so excited he was finally gone, and I would not have to be around him again. Not more than a couple days later I saw him walking to the front door and wanted to run and tell my mother to run. She said it's okay, he was drunk and allowed him to come back around. After all of that she took him back and said she loved him, and it will be okay. I was so angry and could not understand why she would let him back in and around us again. I would ask the moon to kill him or take us away from this place. Never did I get a response, but I knew I had to do something. I wanted to kill him and was going to try. The next night my grandmother and aunt showed up and was talking to us about the situation that happened, and I told my grandmother I was going to kill him. She looked at me with such confusion and my aunt looked scared. Why would he say that they asked? My mother replied he do not like being punished by him for doing bad things. Korey is a troublemaker and causes all kinds of problems and needs to be punished. I was so mad she lied and stood up for this man. I just wanted to scream at her and tell them everything, but the moon was full and called my attention. I could not stop staring at it. I was hypnotized by it and just watched it and faded away from the conversation.

I let it go and went in for the night. Then I woke in the middle of the night to feeling someone putting a hand on my chest. I woke up and looked around but could not see anyone in the pitch black of night. I could feel someone looking at me. As I lay there, I could start to see a figure like a shadow and thought it might be one of the men who came over to sleep and was checking the bed to find a place to lay down. I said, "I'm sleeping here you can take the couch; no one is on it."

No answer and no movement. I just laid there and wanted to hear or see something. It was standing still and would not make a sound and I started to get chills through my whole body. Then from my mothers' room a light turned on and she walked out to use the bathroom. As she opened the door and the light shined out into the living room where I was asleep, there was no one standing out there in the area I seen the shadow silhouette. My whole body was frozen still. I did not know what just happened and tried to convince myself I was dreaming and tried to go back to sleep before my mother turned off the light again.

All that night I felt scared and could not figure out why I felt the way I did. My body was feeling so many different sensations and I started to feel like my skin was full of static. I did not know what was happening but after a while I faded to sleep and woke up to the usual day again.

I did not know what to tell anyone or ask if they knew what that may have been. I remember the stories of the skin walkers and the spirits that roam the area. The aliens that everyone would talk about and the lights we would see during dusk and during the night.

Each night after I remember seeing eyes and small figures moving around in the apartment and outside while I would be sitting by myself or walking the trails in the woods. I asked some of the kids in the area and would be called 'crazy' or 'insane' so I stopped telling anyone and kept it to myself.

FOURTEEN
CHRISTMAS SURPRISE

With this man still in the apartment, still picking on me every time I was around, training me to go steal and take from others, if I were not being beaten, I was okay with what he would have me do. I knew it was Christmas time for all the lights and people talking about it, but I knew my mother could not buy us anything for she would say it all the time.

"Do not expect anything from me," she would say. "You better hope Santa is in a giving mood to give to you for all the trouble you cause, you will be lucky to get coal."

I did not try to cause trouble but was always blamed for something I never knew I did. One night I will never forget, was the cold night the front door had a hard knock. There were a special way people would knock so we would know if it was the police or not. My mother's boyfriend ran to the room and closed the door and my mother told me to go look. I opened the door and there stood so many faces cold and fully wrapped up.

"Merry Christmas," they said and handed me a bag bigger than I stood tall.

Full of gifts and presents it was, and my excitement built to my head. I did not know what to do and how to react, so I said thank you and started to close the door. They started singing and said just wait as everyone came to see what is going on? I moved the bag off to the side and watched as they started to sing us a song.

Faces smiling and happy to give, this church close by knew we were poor. We thanked all the men and women who came and for all the gifts they brought us from Santa I was told. So happy I was and excited I felt finally I get to have something of my own. After they left and he came out of the room. I was pushed to the side and was told to sit down let us see what we have in store. Everyone got to open and go through what we got, and I was handed things they did not want and was last to receive and last to be given what no one else wanted.

No matter to me, a gift was a gift, and the love I felt meant so much. I remember I got shoes with batman on the sides and socks no one else could fit. One fake gun and another small toy but my favorite was a teddy bear everyone tried to throw away. I saved him from the trash and sat him next to me and told him I would be his friend. They all laughed and made fun of me, but I did not care for I felt so special and happy. I slept in those shoes and with my new friend and named him after the boy who saved me. Josh was his name and I would tell him everything. Sometimes they would hide Josh from me and make fun of me for getting mad when they did. I remember thinking about killing anyone who tried to steal him or when they would throw him outside. I would hide Josh if I were to go play or have to leave the hose so nothing bad would happen to him.

I am so thankful for everyone from the church that gave me all those gifts and I would go up to that church and they would let me eat when they had pitch-ins when everyone would bring food. They always sent me home with a plate to go. I love those people and the families who knew what I had to go back to and would tell me it will be okay, and you do not have to be like them if you choose. The preacher's daughter liked me and would tell me how she prayed I would be okay. The Sundays they did not see me, she said they would worry but always checked on me when they could. For the first time since my father I felt people cared for me and wanted to help. Later I found out the people at that church knew about my mother, and the daughter heard about me from friends around the neighborhood. Maybe they could help me get ahold of my father so he could come get me and take me away from this life. I felt I was able to get out one day.

Reflection

Living in this lower lifestyle and wanting a handout would be a main program that has to be broken in a major way. Though this was the best thing that could happen to me during this time. My mother and her friends would go into detail on how these people should give us more and do more to support people like us. We cannot have the things they have, and we are not able to buy those things. Not from trying but from not wanting to try.

They knew if we looked poor and could make others pity us, and want to help so they feel better about them self's for being able to have the things to give. They would tell stories about what all they would get for free and what all they would take from the people who would sometimes give or try to share. If they could tell the people had more to give by the clothes or shoes people would wear, they would tell deeper stories on how they were able to get more by telling them lies about a struggle they are going through. Laughing and making it look okay to do this when a child sees this, they will retain and the information and later in life will have this false template that this is life and how they are supposed to live.

I never liked the way it made me feel and I was able to look at them differently from most others around me. I did not want their attention, I just wanted to not be beaten or hurt for not going along. I was told during this time to be a part of them or be thrown out. There was no choice while so young.

FIFTEEN
SCREAMING BLOOD

I awoke hearing my mother screaming at the top of her lungs. We all jumped out of bed and turned the lights on as she opened her bedroom door. Her face was covered in blood as she walked out of the room holding her head. Black liquid ran down her face and as it would dry you could see the stain of oxygen enriched red blood. Her face in sheer terror and pain she stumbled forward screaming for help. All three of us kids are trying to guide her out the door.

    She could barely walk after being beaten and her head getting split open from an ashtray being smashed across her skull. I grabbed her hand and guided while I told my oldest to run across the street and call 911. My sister was screaming and yelling for help and trying to get anyone around. The man who did this was following laughing and yelling if you do, I will kill you. If you call, I will cut your throat in front of them. I looked for a knife and he only had pants on with no shirt or shoes. Nothing in his hands and no belt. So, I knew he left the knife back at home since his blade was in a case next to the bed where he kept it at night.

    He ran up next to us and was telling her to hurry up, come on, the phones right there. Touch that phone and see what happens. Looking into his face with such enjoyment about what he has done. The thrill of causing pain and fear into a drunk, weak female. Not paying any attention to us kids, my sister screaming, people looked out and by the time we got to the phone my brother had 911 on the phone and she told them where they were. He sat on a bench waiting for the police with such a grin on his face.

He would tell her, "When I get out, I am going to fucking kill you. You're fucking dead you stupid bitch." Every time he would say it, I could see the way the pain and fear would cut into my mother. I could see on her face the depth of the words from this man. How it hurt her more than the split skull had put her through.

Just as he was put in handcuffs, he told her three more times how she was a dead bitch when he gets out. The officer told him to shut his damn mouth and you need to learn how to talk to women and grow the fuck up. She can send you away for a long time. He looked right at her and told her to try it. See what happens. I never felt the type of evil and pure hate this man held inside. The darkest soul and the most hate for everyone and everything.

The whole town hated him, and no one wanted him around. The whole town wanted him to go away and my mother told them she loves him. "I love him," with blood on her face and tears in her eyes. The officer tried to explain and help all he could, but she did not want to press charges and allowed us kids to live through this lesson with what was most important to her at that time.

I sat outside for days and nights trying to know why and how this could have happened. Why was she unable to see, feel or understand what we are going through and there were so many options on the table for us. My dad, her mother, other friends of the family, not to mention all the business and working-class men I seen love my mother and ask her to be his all over town.

I started to hold everything in and this darkness inside for the hate I would hold towards this man who had her under his spell. His evil ways and the things he would do to her, but she loved him. "I love him," she would say as if that is all that mattered. All that she cared about. All she wanted was this man and this life of pain and sorrow. The life I would have to see as normal. Every day I was afraid and ready to fight for my life and fight to survive. I was told you are nothing and never will I make it past 18. You are a bad piece of shit kid and no one wants you around. You are a bastard child, and no one will miss your little ass. You would be raped and killed within three days lock up. The same story he would tell me two or three times a week and how he would get in my face and the grim look is burned into my memory.

My world during this time was a dark place and full of constant pain and fear. Every time there was a conversation, everyone one would compete with negative stories. Instead of talking about what they had going good for them, they would engage in conversations with who had the worst experience and who had done the worst in the streets. Who was the eviler man or women and more bad ass? Who did the most damage and who was the wanted by the law the most? Who has the most warrants and if they get caught who has the most years to serve? I would hear them tell stories of what they did to other homes, cars and what they sometimes did to the men, women, and kids in the home if they had to, or wanted to.

There was a level of dense energy and dark intentions from the darkest places of the mind the human conscious could go. They wanted to feed off the weakest. They did not want to even work to steal from others. These cowards would steal from people they would call friend, or from people who were working class, but could not afford much, but would have nice things. I would see them for who they really are. On dark lonely nights, drinking alone and talking to themselves, I could hear these evil men crying, smacking and punching themselves in their own face. "Why did you do that? Why do you make me do this? I do not like living like this. I do not want to be like this anymore."

These men, these grown men would talk to voices in their head and talk to no one next to them late at night when they thought I was asleep. Him sitting on the couch or in the kitchen sitting alone in the dark. Half-awake, still asleep they would say some of the strangest things. Voices and sounds from these men and boys I was around. Drunk or took something I was not allowed, they would talk about what they would see and the things that would happen, to them and to the others in town. Stories of the shadows that would talk to them and the creatures they would see.

Sometimes they were animal like and others they would be Native American women naked and beautiful. They would never finish the story and would be afraid of talking about it. Only when they were drunk or on drugs would they be open about it.

The one thing I felt was weird was when they were sober, or not as under the influence they would look me in the eye and say, "You don't want to know what is out there and what you cannot see. I can see what you and others do not have to see and believe me you do not want them to see you." These men and brothers of mine had been haunted by something and was afraid of whatever it was.

I simply thought of it as what they called in, not what was controlling them. Now I have a better understanding of why they were open to the darkness and why they were also tormented and pushed to be fueled by hate and negativity. Open to what they never knew they could change and ask for help with. Finding in themselves what they needed to change if they genuinely wanted to be different. I think not knowing any other life and only being known for the bad things they have done; they could not forgive themselves.

I now look at who raised them and to the men I never got to meet, but to the stories they told. Beaten everyday if their parents and family saw fit to give them a beaten for this or that. It was always how they worded the phrase. Give them a beaten because they felt like doing it. Sounds like parents that wanted to take anger and stress out on those weaker and closest at the time. I knew a lot of them come from the old west and to look at the years their parents were also raised, you could see the times and the hardships they got raised in and around. I see the process and how there was a broken chain of love and only pain to try to numb away. From one to the other, father and mother, both have habits learned. From years of conditioning and habit, the reaction becomes the tactic to project what the issue or blockage really is.

So, each lesson done to me was them trying to release the pain they might have felt once in their life. The beatings and bashings, the wiping and lashings. So much more of the story to unfold. Reminded I was, almost every time, the words, "Boy you do not even know. I'll tell you what boy, that day you will know that God is not coming to save you."

The words so deep, and the pain you could see on the face of the man as he would tell you it's true. What happened to me was my test and trial to see if my mind would break and my balance working to tip the scale. Even when I tried to get out and get away I could not, I was to go through these lessons so I could experience what I was meant to.

From the beginning I was shocked into this life from dream to reality from that first gun shot. The understanding of who I am to who, and where I stand in this family of shadows and souls. The flame to ground me down, and the mindset to survive and observe what was to come.

Learning to adapt and know that you are owed nothing but can work for anything, means you must be willing to grow. Find your way out instead of seeing yourself locked in. What path to take and what road to go down? Times might get tough, and the path may not be so clear, but you will make it, I promise. If you keep trying you cannot fail.

From the pain I remember and the lessons I have learned, it keeps me happy to see that I no longer live with that energy.

How men would act, and girls were raised is such despair.

The fears that come from the feeling of creating a reality by speaking the words that cut deep into someone's soul.

Hold space for those people and life can change in so many ways.

The trials I have survived, and the lessons of pain made me understand how life gets and what kind of people there are in this world. The energy I lived in and around the men who taught me, was just doing what they thought life was about, and they had no one to show them differently.

So, the lesson of who they are is to see what they were subjected to. The same, if not worse, and the drugs they would take and the state of mind that their parents or kin they were raised with during their times. If I were to erase these memories, I would not know what I know now. So, if you wanted to unlearn what you have learned from these times in your youth, it would be simple to unlearn that this is normal and see it as a bad time in your life, stuff you don't want to hold on to.

Your intention could be simply 'I see this, and I am addressing it'. Then declaring that you are detaching from this and will release your energetic attachment and can see it as a good lesson instead.

If you are triggered by something someone else projects, know what it is from. Ask the question out loud and quieten the mind. You will be able to just know. Run through the memories and see what you want to keep and say what you do not. You can tell your mind what to see and how to feel. Heal the past by allowing it to be understood and released. You only hold on to what you do not fully understand. The question is, what do you bury under feelings and emotions? Allow yourself to feel and address the emotions and remove the suppressed feelings so you can move on. Know what it is like to not have that blockage or trauma that keeps you from living your truth.

I was not to be removed, and I was to see so I could help so many others later in life and hold space for whoever relates. I survived during this time to understand the people and teachings for what was to come later in life so I can help others learn from all of this. All the training and lessons would come to serve me as these men knew my fate. All the anger and hate would prepare me for what was to come after all that had been learned, just from being around home. My world was about to change, and many new things would have to be learned on the fly and on the go.

These first two years are still not done for it was time to learn about going to school. The stories and tales I would hear from others, school was a place where I would make new friends and learn even more.

What dreams I would dream and fantasies I would think about this heaven outside of this hell. The things I will see, and the time I will share, like a fairy tale story I've heard. So mysterious it was, life inside of these places where children and adults all go. What will I do, and what can I learn, with so many questions and doubts?

SIXTEEN

THE CABINS

The cabins, like many throughout the mountain towns in Arizona were made shack, and barn style homes. Who needs electricity when you have fire or candles? Wild men and women who lived to be free and, in a way, they thought they were condemned to as well. Proud of the life they choose to live, yet angry about it all at the same time. Happy to have a small home with power and a water heater to wash clothes and bathe. If you had a TV and power, you had it good and attracted all the young ones in the area.

Us kids would play in herds from age group to age group. As kids do, we would wake up early and eager to start the day; wake up, get out, or go to school. The adults would yell if we made noise, so if you were off or you had no school, it was getting out and not making a noise until others wake up. If you disturb any of the men while they sleep in the community, he is libel to shut you up quickly by knocking you out, slapping you down, or just punching you in the chest.

Older brothers and sister did the same to whoever was younger and smaller. What they were taught, they would remind all of us smaller and younger kids to do the same and keep quiet and out of the way.

As in the animal kingdoms the Alpha would always set the frequency of the group and what the plan was for the day. For all the males who wanted to compete and see who was worthy of a challenge. The men ready to see how tough you are always, waiting and watching to try to catch you slipping (not paying attention). If you are in this community, you'd better know how to fight, or you will not survive. If you wanted to act like or talk like an adult, you will be treated as such. Learn your place in the pack or you will be discarded. If you become a problem to the pack, you will be warned once and then the example will be made of you and what you did. Adapt quickly of fall behind.

Know where you are going by remembering where you have been. Keep track of large landmarks that you can see from a long distance. Place it in your mind and always know where it is in your mind. So, no matter how many times you get turned around, if you can see the landmark, you will know where you are. Learn the stars and keep your cardinal directions in the sun and night sky. Learning the stars and consolations would fascinate me and I would always ask about life out there and would wonder what all was possible. I had many conversations with many different people about life outside our planet. From working class men and women, bikers, mountain men, adults in the neighborhood, and native Americans on the Navaho reservation just outside of town. I would listen to all the stories and tales about the people and creatures out there in this dimensional universe. We are one of many I was told. I was told of the creation myths and legends of the skin walkers and shape shifters in the mountains as well as the animal spirits in the wild; How to call to them and ask for help. If you need questions answered or help understanding anything, all you need to do is look to the sky and ask for the answers. Listen inside and connect with what is out there in the stars that is meant for you. You will just know and feel you know. Also, family is who you feel is family. Do not let anyone tell you family is only blood related. I was drilled with this every day in so many shapes and forms. My sister, brother, cousin, uncle, mom, dad, and code names to try to keep up with. Everyone was one of those names but had nothing to do with blood or marriage. Depending on the age group of the individual and the sex/gender? Boy=brother, bub, bro. Girl=sister, sissy, sis, and so on. I was seeing how families grow quickly when you get down to your community.

No matter the disagreement with, and of your kin, they are and will be all you have. You are responsible for your family. Give everything you can if you have enough to share with your family. Take in your family if you have the room and they are in need. If you do not help your family when they need something, and you are able to give them what you have but do not. You will be taken advantage of and they will rob you just as if you were someone they do not know or care about. They will take from you anyway. There is a thin line between everyone, and you are only part of the family if you have something to offer, or there is a mutual agreement or understanding.

The rules often changed during times of who held the title 'Head of household' and both would fight about it. Men and women would fight and argue and many times blood would be shed. These women in love with these wild men had their own set of rules and conditions. Many times, the police arrived guns and lights in hand. Doors kicked off their hinges, "Stop! Freeze!" and listen to what they say. "Hands on your head and slowly walk backwards," as they guided us where to go.

Placed in cuffs and treated like a criminal or like an animal. The public beatings and punishment for not listening or not moving quick enough as the police wanted you to. Humiliated and made examples of daily during the confrontations between my people and the police. The police treated us like criminals every chance there was, making it a point to slow down and check us out or follow us to where we would go. It was as if they knew where the trouble came from and who to look at, but by treating us kids like criminals, they will not stop a kid from acting like one.

There would be so many conversations about how my brothers would try to get jobs and work, but couldn't since they are from the ghetto; and people in town know their parents and who all they hang out with, no one wanted to give them a chance. It would make them become what others see them as since there was nothing they could do to change the mind of the people in the town, or the police. So, from teenage years and under, we were seeing that we were being watched and hated for what the men and older boys and girls do from the neighborhood we lived in.

It added to the programming that we are a product of our

environment and adds to the blockage of seeing any way out. Since the only fun we could have was to run from the cops for chasing us, for questioning and checking us for drugs, we would see it as a game of always getting away with whatever we want, and the worst the crime, the bigger the thrill.

It does take more than just environment to persuade an individual to do the things they do. When it is your entire world, in a neighborhood of the same kind of people, you do not have a choice but to learn the hard way. This will not make you weaker. This will not make you know better. This will be what will, or will not, hold you back from being what it is you want to be, or have what you want to have.

Now, to the people who think this makes you stronger for learning the hard way, it is harder to break a hardened path beaten into what you think your path should be. When it comes time to submit to the universe, and to your purpose in life, you will have a hard time committing to the path that you have to trust and believe is there. Learning the hard way only makes it easier to see the ways not to do something. Lessons are lessons at the other end of not knowing.

Every night there was always a fight or issue, and if the moon was full and able to show, it was time for a party. Fire and ice, with beer in disguise covered by a cloth or a bag. If anyone disagreed or liked opposite, then the other they would settle by a throw down show. Guns, knives or knuckles, the choice was open for discussion and they would engage in settling the score. Throw down any weapons and get in the open and see who is ready to go. Younger boys would try to show off, and lessons they would learn about not being ready. Also, the older men would decide for the younger boys and the older men would call them out and they had no choice. It is time to fight if another man wants to test you and is ready. Each of us kids had no choice and where picked off at random. Each young man that would be picked off, would take what had happened to them the night before, such as getting into a fight and loosing, out on us smaller and younger kids; this way we would not see them as weak. Many times, we were picked on for seeing them crying, or in pain and they would take their anger and pain out on us smaller kids, boys, and girls. Beaten and bruised, but the hurt was not from a wound but the pride they felt. You could see it in his face as the younger boy would smash my face into the floor and punching me while I was down. They would release their own pain from being the smallest in the room at the time. The younger boys wanted to cause someone else pain from the pain he felt inside.

Public humiliation, not always deserved, but projected for the older men, as they did not like the younger men. For the music, lifestyle, and colors of the other bandanas started to not agree and one did not understand the other; bikers and outlaw's, mountain men, and drivers, so many different choices and groups. Family's started to divide and people from outside the neighborhood would come in and get removed or carried off bloody and beaten if it were needed.

Learning how to fight, how to move in and out, what to do when fighting in each fighting style; how to counter and defend from the fighting styles taught by ex-military and prison convicts, with Kung fu trainings and fighting skills.

Some of the brothers in the neighborhood taught me about energy and what they called the force. How we can control our body with our mind and how to train it to become one with the body. This was my ninja training and shadow work becoming one with nature and healing my body with my mind if wounded. How to stretch and work the fluids through your body and what exercises are best for the human body.

With all the different skills and knowledge, I was surrounded by I was driven to learn everything I could from everyone I was around. The more I knew, the better I could be, and the more I would be able to accomplish. This was a way for me to learn what I could so I would be able to get out of this life and do what I felt I was here to do. I needed to master how to live in a place where evil and hate meets in one destination to see what happens each night.

Witches and spells, crystals, and tales, for the gods and spirits are all around. The stories I would hear, and the spells I would watch, whilst hiding in the shadows of trees. Watching the ritual and hearing intentions, I never fully understood. Not from not listening, but what was the witch seeing? As a child, I could see what she felt. Her emotions and feelings from her singing and screaming the sound I felt to my bones. I see in the shadows what I thought was a man, but I was unable to focus from the candle lights glow. These women would come and go and I would only know they were around or doing rituals when I would see then walking through the woods or during the night seeing their campfire on top of the hill.

This place was dense with low energy and my malnourished mind was surrounded by fear and anger. I was open to the wrong energy and surrounded by angry energy. This is when I started to see things that would scare people to their core. I was told to stop telling people why I cannot sleep, why I would wake up at night screaming, and how I would wake in the night and find myself outside standing in the field behind our cabin.

The stars and the moon light would call my attention and the lights in the night sky as they would go by. My sister would also wake up outside to look for something she could never find. Shadows and whispers with strange feelings, like being watched, and as if someone were standing behind me. I would ask the witches and warlocks these questions and others who I would meet, as well as the natives when I would see them around. If I had questions, they would tell me to ask the shadows what they want? "If you see something, you can ask what they want or what they need to move on. It might be for you to learn something, or it might be for them to learn something."

I was not confused. I felt I understood everything they would say, but still try to figure out having a conversation about talking to shadows. They would talk as if they knew what I was seeing and how to remove them or communicate with them. The ones who knew what I was seeing and dreaming told me I was special and since they are coming to me, I needed to listen and learn. I was told, "They do not sense evil or dark energy from your energy," so I was told I may be getting visited by watchers and messengers. I was told how to request help and speak to them directly; and how to see with my mind's eye.

I was not able to speak or move during the night when it would happen or sometimes during the day while walking through the woods. I would wake in the night and be perfectly still, unable to move. I would feel sore the next day and have marks on my body. There were a few others that would have this issue and was willing to talk about it. There would be feelings and dreams that felt real, and some was as if it happened but there was no way to be sure. Some of the nights when there was a lot of drugs going around, and it was just before dawn, I would see people sit up or get up and do the strangest things as if they were a puppet. From sitting on the kitchen counter, opening, and closing cabinet doors, then back to sleep to sexual acts while next to or over others sleeping. I have had to act asleep a few times during these acts and they would speak in mumbles and sounds, not words I understood. When I would ask about it to other people, they would tell me I am lying, or I am crazy. The Indians told me they were possessed with a dark spirit and to stay away from the ones I see do that. They would walk naked over me sleeping on the floor and rubbing their hands all over their body and sexually pleasing themselves while standing in a room full of sleeping people. They would sometimes finish by having sex with whatever man she woke up by oral stimulation, even if his girl or wife were next to them sleeping. I witnessed first-hand how the rules of love and lust played out every day.

The young girls would be abused and taken advantage of during these years of struggle while living in the cabins. When the mothers and working women would go to the store or working together, they would leave us kids with the men, older boys, and girls. The older kids would run off and leave me and the youngest stuck around these dark and animal-like men.

The young girls would be made to, or would offer sexual acts, so they would get drugs or for money. If they wanted something, they would have to "earn it" was the phrase. The stories the young girls would tell me crying and saying if I tell anyone, they will kill her and me. They were not alone in this sharing and many of the girls would tell me what, and who would do what to them. I got used to the fact the girls and friends would always feel comfortable telling me, knowing I would never tell or put them in a situation they would suffer from. In return they would try to do to me as they were taught to do to the men. I would ask them why they wanted to do that to me, and they would say so they could know the difference and try to understand. Wanting to show their affection and being forced to is a different energy completely. These young girls were told that if they do this for their men or for the men they like, then they will never have a man stay with them. So even though this evil is happening to these young girls they are being told if you do not find a way to like doing what men want from you, then you will be cheated on and alone. The mothers are telling how their father left her for a dick sucking whore and the young girls is now programmed that if you do not do that he will cheat. As young girls they are forced to give oral sex to older men threatening to kill her if she says anything. Then secretly trying to find a way to cope with giving oral sex to a man she likes, so she can keep him while having trauma from the action in the first place, battling the emotions obtained from the mother who hates the father.

This might be strange to some to try to comprehend but to kids in this life, and those around these people. these were the only times we knew how to show love for one another. I know brothers and sister who had to do other things for the men and the mothers in the town and neighborhood, but this does not stop only for them. Boys had a choice to survive if they knew what was good for them, they "best just play along". Us young boys would be called toys and were told "come here and do what I say". Alone and high while still drunk from last night, they would play with what they wanted. What we had to do was whatever the neighbor women would say because if you don't, she will tell everyone you tried to fuck anyways while she was asleep, and she had to stop you. They tell you they will kill you without thinking about it. They would tell us they wanted our energy and to "taste the taboo flavor of our soul".

Calling out names and language, moaning and groaning, and they do what they feel compelled to. Each would have their own experience and it was hard to make sense of what some boys had to do. It was erotic and some of the boys enjoyed what they got to do. The younger girls would sometimes have to watch and sometimes help or join in.

The things we would see, and life here was open to whatever the night would call for. We would have to learn how to slip away when we could, and then we would take what we would learn and play with the others from the same community in the woods, or just out back in the field during the night. So many stories I remember going through in this community and around the town. This was not just in my community, but the whole town had stories. People would do things that could make you sick. You must do what you must survive or what you think you must, because what other choice do you have as a child? Afraid and with no one to go to, what do you think others would say if you told anyone?

There was a few that tried; and afterwards, the kids were accused of lying, the parents got them back and there was hell to pay; some of the kids committed suicide. I was losing friends and having to try and keep kids from talking about themselves. Many aged five to six years old had already decided to die by listening to other kids wanting to die, just as I have felt many times before. This was not just in the rougher side of town either. I heard stories from all sides of town and from neighborhoods you would not believe something like this would happen in.

I would learn more about people and other households and what all would go on with others. At first, I wanted to go to school to get away and to meet new people so I might be able to get out. A single father that likes my mother and will help give me a better chance at life, or another family to take me in. It was nothing like I thought it would be, and was the reality of what I needed to face that would push me over the edge.

I would become what they wanted while living with the people I was with, and how I had no other choice but to get along so I could go along. Nobody understood when I would get into fights and must defend myself. Kids would make fun of the way I would smell and how I had lice. I was unwanted from the first day of school.

I heard the teachers talking about how they need to sit me away from the other children and told the other children not to sit with me or play with me.

Do you know what it is like to be called lice boy at school for your first experience and have all the kids point and say mean things?

This new place I was told I would get to learn and do fun cool things, and instead I was hated and pushed to the side.

My family and all the people I were living around had a reputation and well-known way of life. I was treated as one of them by default, and no matter how hard I tried to do better or learn how to change, the universe had different plans for me.

In school I would stab kids with pencils and pull their chair out from under them while leaning forward on the table so they would drop and hit their chin on the table. One kid was sticking his tongue out at me and I smacked up on his chin so he would almost bite it off. I would laugh and make it like I thought it was funny and as if I liked to hurt other people. Children started to fear me and when they fear me, they no longer make fun of me, or try to hurt me. After that I wanted to be the most violent so people would stop being mean to me and just be afraid of me.

Some girls liked that about me, so it added to the fun of showing off and acting stupid to get the attention. I now see what the men who raised me did to program me and to prepare me to deal with these challenges while going to school. They must have gone through something similar when they were young. Each day there was a fight or someone challenging someone else or fighting over girls. Even if she liked another boy, they would fight for the right of the girl but sometimes the boy she liked would loose and then it was a whole episode of drama.

Looking back now I can see all the TV shows and remakes of the episodes our parents went through and had projected on to the kids. Complaining about the divorce or separation and talking about it to your kids and while your kids are young. In the house around the energy, they would pick up the energy frequency you are telling in the story. Everyone does not pay attention to the programming of youth while they see and feel what the parents are going through.

You do not have to be involved or in on the fight, you can just feel how your parents feel about each other.

Just the same as when you are close to someone you can feel when they are hurt or angry. Kids would have movie star problems and fights to go through similar stories that their parents went through or told them about. I kept it simple and tried not to side with either one, and instead I would look from both sides and give my opinion. I was not one to have many friends and so I only heard about the game's kids would pay. I put fear into others so no one would know how I felt and so no one could use this against me. I can now see it was how much they hated themselves and would want to look at other people and other problems so they would not have to look at their own stories.

Sad and lonely how mad they are for being judged for something in the same way. For me back then it was power over others. I was over being picked on, and now I am going to scare you all. I wanted to be so bad that my mother's boyfriends would fear me. I knew I wanted to train and become what they could never be. The ultimate Alpha no matter where I stand. I would outthink anyone who was bigger, older, stronger, or able to hurt me. I would find ways in and out of any situation and always keep a discipline of personal values and honor, so I would keep the respect of the people in the street.

I would listen to the old schoolers and cowboys in town. Stories of John Dillinger, Bonny & Clyde, Babyface Nelson, Machine Gun Kelly, Pretty Boy Floyd, Al Capone, and the stories of the Chicago, Los Angeles, New York, and Mexico gangs and mafia. For hours I would listen to them tell how they would run from the law and how to keep a low profile from the government. What to do about rules and how to honor them. Lessons learned from other failures and what not to do; Criminal Grooming 101 with a mix of Wild West outlaws. Outlaws would always tell me I had "an old soul". They would always say "there is something about you, you act older than you are", "The way you understand what I am saying, and I can tell you feel what I'm saying", "I know you are going to do well". The phrases "just remember, and do not you ever forget" are things I heard a lot. I was told if I can see the world for what it is and accept what is happening at that moment to be just what is happening, it is not how it is; That there is nothing that can make you do anything, but what you think of it in that moment and what you let it make you feel like. The feelings you give to any reactions attached to emotion to something you remember in your mind. This is only happening in the way you feel it is happening. No matter what It is you must do always remember you control if it will be a negative or positive response.

I never really knew who this man was, or what he was always saying, but he would be around here and there. Nobody seemed to mind him or mess with him. He was a large older man and he would always make sure the kids where okay. Telling someone they need to "quit while you're ahead" and "grow up quick or you're done", was another one of his sayings. He was a tumble weed he would say. I just roll with the wind. I was always looking to see what I could learn from him and from all the older men that would come and go. Anyone who had something to teach or something I could learn from I would be around asking questions. No video games or friends to distract me, all I would do is find something to learn. My education was from who I was around and not from the schoolbooks or classes I would be made to go to.

At school, the response to any questions I had was of others not trying to be close to me from the smell of my clothes and that I had lice. They also did not like me to get too close to their desk or too close to their personal items. Making me check my pockets before I could leave class. "Stand there, empty your pockets, show me what is in your hands?" They would look at what I had, and sometimes even ask me if what I was holding was mine or if I had stolen it. At school, the teachers would not like to get close to me and would sometimes cover their nose from the smell of unwashed clothes, sweat, fire pit, and cigarettes.

Our mothers would steal from Walmart and other small stores. We would learn to do the same if we wanted new clothes. We would steal and get in trouble for it, but they would steal they would say they are allowed to; they are adults. Sometimes if we stole something for them as well, they would not tell use to not do that. They would take advantage of us kids stealing and taking from others as well. Teaching us to get what we want by stealing and not earning it with work or service. My mother thought the world should give to us poor people. They should give and supply us with work and supplies. They would put it in our head that we are innocent for taking from others who would not appreciate it like we would. If they treat it like its nothing in our opinion, then we will take it and enjoy it for you. Take what you want in this life I would be told and cheered on. No one will give you a helping hand, and the world will try to take all you are worth or wants you to die if you do not submit to the government. Angry and sad most of them would use sexual desires to numb the pain and emotions of their own memories. When you add drugs and alcohol at the same time, there is going to be things you see happen as a child in that environment. You just must walk away and know when you need to be the adult and separate yourself from what they are going through. Late at night, middle of the day, it did not matter. When they were ready to take it from the women or girls, be ready for the wild west show for all to see. If you did not want to watch go away or look the other way. Older man and women, older man and young girl, older women and young boy, young boy, and young girl, young girl, and young girl and yes there was stories of boy and man and so on. This was not a place of just a few people here and there. This was everyone had something with at least one other. Day after day, and night after night, sleeping for only a few hours.

We would get stopped walking down the street and checked by the police in the town because they all knew who we are and where we are from. They would ask where the weapon is, or where are the drugs as they pointed their guns at us. Spot check or arrested if you stayed to get questioned and they always would ask who was in town? What men are hiding in the cabins? Where are they keeping the stash? We all knew better and would say the same thing, "What are you talking about?"

They would push and shove and sometimes put their gun in our mouths and say are you sure you want to lie? They would push and shove and punch you in the ribs knocking the air out of them. The police would also make them cry from the pain and then make them walk through the neighborhood crying so everyone could see. They also liked to try to humiliate us and see if they could make us break down and feel stupid.

When we would get home and tell the others what happened and who they asked about, we would get beaten again. "What did you tell them? What did you say? I will fucking kill you if I find out you said anything."

We did not tell if we were questioned or stopped for fear of the trial you would face. You were then called a snitch deemed a narc and brutally beaten and sometimes never seen again. There is always someone watching and if you found out one of the boys or girls got stopped and questioned and did not report it, you were cast out of this crew and all other avenues are cut off due to if you withhold information, you are hiding something.

Harbor anyone you're considered a narc, or a snitch and you will be treated as such. Stand in your truth and take the consequences. As you need to prove who you are and where you stand each day you are alive and live around these people.

Know your chain of command and do what the adults say to do for your life depends on every choice you make every day. These men would put us through tests and trials as well as send us on missions testing our skills and loyalty.

The girls would be treated different of course, and if he wants something from her, she gives it willingly or he will take it unwillingly.

If a woman tells you to come here, you seriously have to the count of three to get over to them and do what they say. I have seen what happens when one decides to say no. He was knocked out and had a broken nose for not doing what one of the mothers wanted and she made up a story about the boy. After all of that he was called humiliating names and rumors spread all over town. She told everyone he tried to rape her while she was passed out on the couch naked. Made the story up and they believed her and of course this story would cause anyone to think in that way when his stepmother was the one accusing.

Who would think in that way and be okay with addressing it? Yet we all knew what was to be true. These men took what they wanted and so did the women. Some wanted more than others and down the rabbit hole they would go. If she wanted to see it or play with it, you had to make sure no one knew and in the end all we wanted was to get through the day with the least amount of pain and suffering.

Looking at what state of mind they were in to do and to crave this kind of energy and taboo rituals of having sex with underage kids. They were in so many layers of false reality and an open channel for all kinds of things to come and go.

The Indian reservation just a walk up the hill had special medicine that would take you places. These people would mix drugs and create new drugs to try out and did this always while drinking. The Apache tribe with their many rituals and customs were not understood to a lot of people. When I would hear the stories of the young Indian girls on the reservation and how they were treated like animals and slaves to the eldest man of the family. I would feel the same about what I wanted to do to them as I did my mother's boyfriend.

Sisters and cousins would tell me how they would be raped by brothers and uncles as well as father in laws. How they would be beat and abused while the men are drunk and angry for no reason. Just the way they would speak about it like this was all there was to life and as if they were dead inside. I would tell them to run away or go to someplace else far away from here. The girls from the Indian tribes would tell me how no one would take them in, and other tribes are not open to taking in each other. These men and boys who did these things to these girls and did it as if this were the way of things, angered me to the point of wanting to tear down the whole town. Watching nothing but suffering and pain while feeling as if I had it easy compared to the ones I would talk to.

Knowing the men and the boys whose teaching help create what they did and how they showed up in life. Numbing reality as a diversion so they cannot see what they do not want to know about themselves. They would distract with beer and sex as well as any hobby to keep their minds busy from the truth. The drugs they would take would always get stronger and stronger or they would take more and more. Things that would make you see outside of this world watching and listen to them as they were on their trip. The voices they would speak to and the visions they would see during these hallucinations. Walls falling, portals opening, and creatures sitting in the room with us. Lights and fairies and so many different journeys and so many different stories were told.

I would watch and sit in these circles and wait until they would be so high, I would be able to get what they were smoking and take a hit of it before they realized it was me. The first time I did it was while we were all inside from the cold. Crammed in one little room body for body, shoulder to shoulder. There was not an empty spot on the floor without a body. Puff. Puff. Pass. Hand it off until they do not realize they handed it to me. Sitting in this room in a black light and full of kids high and talking about the universe and all its mysteries you would probably start to see the things like I did to. When you're open to it and you look for it. It will be open and look for you.

Nighttime in the mountains on a clear night and you will see all kinds of things. Depending where you are, you can see stars, planets, and the milky way. In an open valley on a clear night you can see so much of the galaxy and stars. The full moon would shine back and light up the night and was the time of rituals. From having drinks to casting spells and the Indians would have their own rituals which most whites were not allowed to see or be a part of. I would watch and was fascinated by the way each would have a different approach but still the same amount of energy. Good or bad. It was the amount of energy they gave to the act or intention. People with love would smile and you could feel the love and sweet smell in the air when preforming a ritual or act with the intention of love and lusting. When the act was for giving and grace, you could feel the connection to the earth as if she were holding you.

During the times of opening to the unknown and being called to open portals and communication with whoever was calling them, was a feeling of fear and adrenaline. My senses were always wild and chilling. I could tell it was because my physical body was not use to the energy, so it received it with a warning sign. I learned the feeling of fear for the negative and fear for the unknown. The difference was that negative would make me angry and the unknown was exciting.

I loved to laugh and smile while being around others affection. I loved so many of the girls and sisters I had around me feeling powered by the love they had for me. I could feel them feel safe and calm in my presence, and love as the brother in the community. I would give all I could and would stand and fight with any of them if needed. I would fight, without question, for any of my brothers and sisters, even if they were in the wrong. I would be there if needed to confide in and to hold if needed. Pain and love were all we had in those times growing up around the men and women we were raised by. We would see men beating the women like dogs and they would scream out, "Do not leave me," if they tried; "I love him and I want him," though he blacked both eyes and busted your skull!? So confused we would be and ask why to our mothers and they said, "One day you will understand what it means to love."

That made each of the kids I grew up with have their own facts and outlook on the word love. Shut the emotions off or you will be consumed by them we were told. If you care for anyone, they will be your downfall and a weakness will not help you survive the life those men lived.

We would see how the women would act while the men were around and how different they seemed while the men were away. They would call them names and hate them when they are gone but when they came back a while in the house, they acted like they were their kittens. Submissive and purred like a kitten when the men would tell them to. The control these men had on their women was like magic or a curse. How could anyone love someone so evil or low energy like the men they would choose. These were who you want to raise and teach your kids?

They would always talk down about school and education, but also tell you to go get out of the house and get education even though you will never succeed. They would teach us about dropping out of school and selling drugs and running guns or leading people through the mountains for money so they can make it out of Mexico.

I have been told stories about how to take money from these families and while in the mountains as they would sleep, they would leave in the night or kill the whole family taking the money and walking away. Selling Native American drugs and alcohol to those who wanted what we had and accepting sexual favors for the exchange. I learned how to barter and trade and how to see quality in what is around. What to steal and where to take it to make money to eat and live as you can.

Survival was a skill trait that is helpful to learn and know but, in my opinion, not the best way to live your life. Some of these people love this life and it is a sense of not being in the system or being a part of the norm. They see themselves as rebels and living the wild west dream as they want and the only way, they see they can. We must remember the people who live this way also think there is no other. They believe this is what they must settle for. No other way out and afraid of trying. They think they will fail if they try any other. Fear of trying and no one to inspire you to change and there is the problem with most in these situations. When you are surrounded by fear and only one or two glimpses of hope, what will be more likely to persuade them to change or stay the same?

This small shack community was a mix of the people everyone would judge and hate for not understanding that most of this life was taught and told that is all they are worth. It would then be said as a distraction that they do not want all the nice things and the big house, while making excuses how that does not make them happy. All I need is this they would say hiding from the truth inside that this is all they believe they are worth. I also would hear the moments of pain and hatred for the life and homes we would live in and must be around: "I wish I could afford this; I wish I were them; I wish I could have that."

I could see that they really did not like who they were choosing to show up as and did want the nicer things in life. I could see they did not want to do the extra work it would take and the effort to keep up on keeping the appearance of the nicer neighborhoods. Each of the cabins was about the same except you could tell only from the theme of the décor in the home. Stones and crystals, relics and wands, fairies, and dragons all over the home. Some would have only bottles of beer and posters of women in bikinis or naked depending on who it was. Some of the cabins in the community, kids are not allowed in and there was a code or a knock you had to know. They would cook drugs and have 'adults only parties' that we did not see or know about. Some of the homes would be a hide out for others that needed to disappear from the law. Not trusting anyone in the community some of the homes were for stashing and trafficking unknowns.

Some of the cabins would have us kids pile in and watch movies if they had a VCR and TV. We would steal movies and borrow others and was the only entertainment we would get. I remember one of my first movies I was able to see was Legends of the Fall with Brad Pitt. The only reason we got to watch the movie so much was because he is almost naked in one part and the mothers and girls would tell how they would bathe him with their tongue and let him put it anywhere he wanted. On and on they would talk about it not knowing us kids are hearing everything they would say. Some of them had pornography and videos we would watch when they were not home or around. Late nights at the bar or at other home parties, and we were left home alone. The older girls would watch and then use me as the lesson and tell me what to do. I would do what they wanted and played all the games, and even later that night outside in the woods. Sex and play were always going on whether with the same or different people. We were never forced to do so with each other, and the adults only knew when someone would get caught and they would tell everyone. Brothers with sisters and cousins from all over, the amount of incest and family that played with each other was just as common as with others. This was known throughout the community but left alone because it was a taught negative frequency that enveloped the community.

Look at what if everyone you know is in this kind of mind state, and everyone you want to tell you want to change, would turn against you as soon as you told them? They would project fear and judgment on you for trying to be better and make you feel bad for trying to leave them.

I would see how many times friendships where broken over the simple color of the gang's bandanna of the neighborhood you lived in or had to move to due to your parents work or affordability. The colors of the gangs and crews on the street, townships and suburban areas coming together against their own neighbors.

No longer were we in this life together but instead we were segregating, separating, and pushing others away. I could not get a friend from the nicer sides of town due to who I was raised by and how no parent wanted their kids to be friends with a bastard child raised by criminals and well known for the bad things I had to do and be a part of. Though I do not hate them for even then I knew they were just as ignorant and did not know any life outside of working more than the time you spend with your family. Dads working overtime. Moms talking to another guy from work. Sister is having sex with a couple guys in the neighborhood and brothers trying to have sex with girls from the same neighborhood. I would hear their parents fighting about, "Who is she calling you this late?" and calling each other cheating bastards and she a dirty whore. I been on a friend's roof top talking to them through their window listening while his parents fight on the back porch, so the kids do not hear. Not knowing we are just above them listening to the whole conversation.

I was good at hiding and blending into the shadows at night and could see clear by moonlight. I was so good I could sneak into people's homes while they were awake and move around undetected. To see friends and girls, and sometimes take food. The conversations I would listen to and the things that would happen when people thought no one was around or looking, let me know what happens when the real side of the human experience comes out. Men and women, young and older, would engage in such discussions as well as fantasies, love, lust, and experiencing life. Questions answered, loyalty tested, and choices everyone had to make. Why don't you love me? Why don't I matter? What is going on? Are we done? Can this be over? I want to die. I don't love you anymore. I am leaving you. I hate you. The reasons come in all flavors as lessons.

I remember the dark sided and the ones people would not want to believe. The stories of the housewife alone at home sleeping with a younger boy so she feels power over someone less than her. The working husband having sex with young girl at work or from the neighborhood for money. How they love each other at night yet have this shadow life. You see there was one life living the story they played along with while another one lived what they felt like doing. To hear this conversation, they admitted the one to the other. Not with who or how, just there has been interaction with another. I knew the girl he was paying, and I was the boy playing with my friends' mother. The husband told the wife to deal with it and stop her games or he will leave her with nothing; "Without me you will be nothing and no one will want you with three kids."

She would ask how to fix this, and the man told her it was simple. Forget about it and keep him happy while never questioning him again or he would make sure she would have nothing and that no one would want her. He then told her to kneel on the porch and now suck him off to prove the loyalty she better has to him for giving her the life she would have never gotten without him. She without question did what he said, and I had to wait until they were done before I could move off the roof so I could get back to the cabins.

Even after all that the mother would still do what she wanted but knew how to hide what it was she was doing. I was let in and allowed to wait for my friend to get back and it started with his sister. The mother-in-law caught us and she was drunk enough to show us and explain what to do and how it works.

Times and days later she would use me, and I could see the energy behind it. The husband was older and liked the young girls and the girls would offer to play for money. The things girls would do for a twenty-dollar bill and how good they were they would tell in full detail. They learned from their own mothers how to do it right or he will go and find another. Girls take on their mother's wounds from what the last man did to her and how he hurt her. "That dirt rat bastard left me for that dick sucking whore!"

Where do you think one of her traumas originate from? If you are not good at it or do this one thing for your man, he will leave you for another. It builds guilt and resentment in the subconscious mind of the young girl or sometimes the only way to feel love or show love. Not saying you both do or do not have to enjoy it. It is in what way your energy is directed at it.

Even boys can get it in their head that if Dad left Mom for a girl who sucks dick better or more often that it is okay to do so. Dad cheated and as we grow older young boys get the same verbal lashing in a different way. "Do not be out there like your piece of shit father cheating around with dick sucking whores." Then wonder why they end up the same way as the father. Parents put their own traumas on their children and so on the cycle goes. The young girls crying to me sitting in the dark under the sky outside away from all the noise going on about what happened. These are the stories we kid share when we are together and there for each other. Only because we all know what is happening all around trying to understand what is happening and how to love in life and do what we can.

Looking back, I try to see not looking at what happened but understanding why it happens in that way. The one you would judge in the situation is a trigger to something you are taught. At the end of it there is a way to see it as if you never heard or dealt with it before. Unlearn what you were taught to think and feel. See it with how was she raised and was she shown the same, and did the man's father do the same and made it okay to do?

I look now and see I had to experience this for some reason for myself but also another. The way people forget what we are all subject to while we are young. The way we felt as a child will reflect as we are older. Our natural state is a childlike energy. When humans have these projected emotions and feeling towards anything else, we have someone else's filter over our eyes. Yes, things are not always the best and greatest but every day we are alive we have a chance to make it work. I was in a place I would not know until later was a place to have the darkest nights so later in life I could receive the most amazing and beautiful days. What happens to us in the past will shape how you see the world ahead. Unlearn these teachings and feel for yourself what is right and what does not serve your best self. I was able to see in all classes of people the world is not what you see others living as. It is what moments in your life do you want to release and what moments do you want to have in the future.

I would ask anyone if they would truly go back, would they? You know you would have to go through it all again in some way or another. I know for some reason this will happen to teach us what we need to see and how to look at the lessons. Who not to trust and how not to hate? We all knew exactly what each parent thought of the other and no matter the situation everyone has their story and version of what happened. These lessons just taught me to look deeper into the eyes and the soul. I can feel inside what you harbor at night from the place I was molded; I have felt that what you feel. So now I see that the feeling to me is for me to hold space for you so you can let go.

We wonder why we attract the friends and people into our lives that match up with your frequency and emotional status. Some friends have such a deep connection until the emotional boundaries are crossed and one moves on and the other resents them for it. We hold on to relationships for fear of change and fear of new. Until we let go of what is not working and try something new that does. You will continue your pattern that you have been taught in some way or another only of what you know of. The things that happen to us, good or bad, leads us to the version you choose to be okay with. Choose who you are, and you can change with just a thought. How do you want them to remember you? Live life and know it is okay to try new things. Lessons to learn and experiences to pass on. What your heart tells you is want will help guide you.

SEVENTEEN
THE CABINS DOOR BUSTER

I was in the living room on the floor sleeping and it was a quiet night for once. The door came off the hinges and the police stormed the front and woke everyone up at gun point. Handcuffed and lined up we all moved around like cattle. Flashlights in our eyes, they were asking so many questions. 'Who' and 'what' is in the home while looking for drugs and guns is just another day in the cabins. I had to use the bathroom so bad and asked if I could use the bathroom or go on the side of the house. Since I was a boy, he stood me on the other side of the toilet while shining his flashlight right at me. Watching to see if I flush anything down the drain as it states in all drug users' home manual. If they try to come in, flush as much as you can, seriously he had to stand there and watch a little boy pull it out and just pee because the people I was raised around!? I had no way out of this life and was treated like a criminal.

My name was on police records at five years young. Some people would be proud of this notion or think this to be bragging rights. This did not hold me down or make me believe I was one of them. It was just something that happened in the past. They treated me like a criminal, but I knew I was only doing what I had to do to survive. I did not like it, but it was so much a part of my daily life I had to. Then once I made it to where I did not have to anymore, I did not steal or take from others.

The police are just following orders and protocol, making sure I did not think about it and I feel bad for the man who had to stand there following orders. That was not in the details of his job description, but he did what he had to.

Some of the officers of the town would treat me like a dog and challenge me with 'the look' to try something or make them feel unsafe in any way giving them the right to arrest or shoot you. Some would try to get in my head and friend me so I would talk or give them a lead. They liked making me stand out by saying thief in the store or gas station if they see me in there. Pointing me out and making me uncomfortable so I would not steal from the store. I hated them for what they did, but I know what they wanted and how they seen me.

They would see me playing with a fake gun I stole from someone and would tell me if I were to point that at them, they would have the right to kill me. Do not ever point anything at them or make them think I have a weapon, or they will have to shoot me. All I would hear from what they would say is that they would kill me as well. So, if I go home, my mother's boyfriend wants me dead and would kill me for bringing the police around and now I am being told by the police that they wanted to kill me as well. What to do? Survive is all I could focus on.

This place during the time that I was there I remember a puppy who was run over in front of us and while his body was flopping around, and man grabbed a big rock and finished him off. He looked back at me and said, "He is not hurting no more." We dug a hole and said goodbye and I felt a piece of my heart leave me. Knowing he would have a better life and would not have to live like we did, and, in a way, he was lucky to not have to live with us. Every day and night no matter what is going on always surrounded by fear and pain.

Some of the girls had kittens and sometimes the men would kill one of the kittens drunk and wanting to destroy something special. I would have to watch while men would try to snap kittens' necks and kill with passion and pleasure. They would count how many times they could break its neck before the kitten would die. 1, 2, 3, they would count out as the kids would scream stop it and please do not. It would disgust me to see this and I hated what they were. I never thought it was okay or liked when they would hurt animals for no reason other than they wanted to hurt something weaker than they to distract what they felt towards themself.

I had this feeling that they would believe when they did that, they would absorb its life energy and be empowered by the actions. I would sit in this feeling of pain and anger and watch them teach this to other kids. I decided no more, and I was tired and over the stories and anger and pain they wanted to put everyone through. So, it was best for me to sit in the shadows and deal with this world I live in apart from them as best I could. Learn from a distance by listening and watching other trials and errors. Running from the police and stealing from each other this game was real, and you could pay dearly.

Men and women both had sexual desires and intentions that would continue the cycle of energy that can hold you back and lessen your light in his world. These trials and lessons are not happening to us but for us in ways many would not understand. To investigate the depth of what had happened, understand it happened and I decided that it will not define me or should it you.

EIGHTEEN
YOUR DECISION TO CONTROL YOUR MIND

See yourself in a way that no one else can change and see yourself as you truly are. To know each choice, you make is of your own decision and it is not for anyone else to judge or question. To know that what you choose for yourself will be the best choice to serve the ones closest to you. Trust in yourself to know what is right with no influence from any other. You do know what is right and what is wrong. At the end of the day, you must live with yourself for the rest of your life. Do you want to live knowing that you choose to do what someone else wanted you to do and determine the rest of your decisions for the rest of your life? These blockages and filters are the only thing holding you from seeing the future and keeps you hiding from your light. The triggers you have and hold to other stories will cause judgement, envy, and hate. While others live their lives as they choose no matter the cost or struggle, or you can live your life through the eyes of others telling you how to live. Dig deep and find more trust in yourself. Look to your knowing not questions you have been conditioned to.

Our natural state is happy and blissful, not someone who is taught pain and hate. Release from the pain and emotions you hold on to and do not let go of what others say, think, or tell you to do. If you need to borrow some of my love and faith that you are stronger and fully capable of letting, go of whatever you know is blocking you, then I give you my love right now to breath in for the count of four and hold for the count of four. Breath out for the count of four then hold for the count of four. Repeat three times and as you breath out on the last breath, just relax and smile for as long as you can. Do not worry I will wait while you take a minute.

Do this quick simple breath anytime you need to get to a place where to need to find a little clarity or to help shift from anger. Repeat as much or if feels right. Make it your own thing. Find a way to take a breath and set intention for when you need it. A breathing technique with your own pace and rhythm. Find yourself and you will be able to remove anything holding you back. During any time, I was going through any of these lessons I would control my breathing and find my physical self-grounded and centered. If I hurt, I would let it hurt and if I needed to release, I would hold and release when I could not hurt others. I would take deep breaths in between beatings and punishment. I could feel my body repairing and starting to be able to control the pain in my body. In the cabins I was beaten and busted up with all the damage in between but never a broken bone or have been casted. I would focus on healing and repairing the body with my mind.

I was trained to hide my fear and to cut off all emotions. I understood how expendable I was, and I mean life or death. Reality was getting through whatever you need too, to survive. Also, whatever is in your way that is keeping you from being the best version of yourself is your own mind. You are what can make you or break you, but every day you are alive and breathing you can change your world. If you need rest, then get rest but do not confuse rest with depression and low vibes. The difference is if you can be honest with yourself and know you are happy to sleep and listen to the outdoors while you nap. Dig down deep and be real as fuck to you and only you can know you. Feel it and let it out with whatever you need to do to let it go. Once you see what it was holding you back you can look form outside and feel. If this is not of your choice to feel and hold back, then you can release any learned pattern. It is okay to know the old ways of family and tradition and so on. Look to the here and now and as your own soul to grow. Work through all patterns you have been taught and see them as lessons as is each to their own. Look as I did as each one a challenge to accepted then overcome and let go.

NINETEEN
THE WOODS

The first time we lived in the woods I remember the excitement I had and how I loved the river cutting through the mountains outside Payson Arizona. There was so much open room to run and climb the hills, the rocks, the trees and the water to cool off in when you need. Fishing and camping with fires burning, cooking hot dogs as the smell comes through the smoke. Trees swaying and laughing birds chirping and dancing. All as the sun peaks at us all down below. The wind and the breeze and the howl of the trees, how the sound went forever it seemed. Then the stars at night and how the moon was so bright and how you could see the face on the moon so clear.

So old and wise did I feel at night just gazing into the moons glare. How small I felt to see the moon and to what I see beyond the stars. What life must be to look at me from whatever I feel is out there. Would they want to know, like I want to know, what it is like where they are from? I wanted the stars to save me and take me away from this place. Beautiful and stunning but the energy I was around was so dark and depressing while everyday stressing. Darkness and evil were the feelings of every night. They never knew what was going to happen or what they were going to do. It is a way of life like the old days in the west on a horse or wagon.

Take all you can to any spot on the river in a place called Flowing Springs. Set up tents or sleep in vehicles if you are lucky to have one. Tarps folded to cover you and to give you shelter and to make sure you have shelter before dusk. Gather firewood and doubled the load for in the morning or if an animal comes in the night looking for food. The rule is if a bear, coyote, mountain lion, wild boar, or wolves come into camp is to get the fire going and make noise. The fire will scare them, and the noise will confuse them while waking others to the uninvited guest. No need to shoot or kill them unless you have to, this is their home before it was ours. This beautiful place, so adventurous and exciting as well as life and death. To live in this place just like the men and women who use to as people who moved west once a time ago. Fetching water from the river for cooking up dinner or whenever you got hungry or needed to eat. Fresh mountain water you could drink from the stream so you could travel the river and survive.

So many days and nights we lived in this life in the mountains of Arizona. Learned the types of trees and the birds to eat but better tasting was the fish. I did not much care for the birds, squirrels, and rabbits the others loved to eat. I loved the water and the fishing but with a fear of the water, I never was shown how to swim. Until one day they had enough of me not swimming and afraid to jump in. So, I was picked up and launched into the river in front of everyone who came to cool off in the river.

My mind reacted and I can remember thinking I was about to die. While in the air I filled my lungs with air and connected to the water and then was engulfed. I tried to hit bottom and launch myself up to the surface but, I was thrown in the deepest part of the cove. Reaching and stretching for anything I could. No one to get me. I remember watching how the dogs would float. I started to mimic the doggy paddle and up I went. Popped up scared and crying swallowing water and choking from all the fear.

By that time, a man grabbed me and carried me to the other side asking me if I was okay? He told them they are stupid, "You dumb asses, he doesn't know how to swim." My people yelled back and challenged him to take his ass on somewhere or keep fishing for an ass whopping.

The man asked if I was okay and told me to walk down to the bridge. Cross where it is safe and take deep breaths, you will be okay. I was able to get out of the situation with learning to doggy paddle when needed and that my mother did not look twice at what had happened.

It was good for me she would say, freely giving permission to anyone who wanted to ruffin me up. Pick and prod and tossed like a doll, they had fun torturing me to the point of wanting to die. So, I learned quickly to wake up early and stay as far out of sight as I could get. Close enough so if they called for me, I could respond or see them, so I was never a target for whatever they wanted to do. I would volunteer to fetch firewood, so I could go out of sight and away to get loads of wood and return. I learned how to cook with ramen noodles and macaroni and cheese.

The boxes of food my mother would go to town for, it was a place they gave to the poor. She would use different licenses and multiple names and say she had more children to support. They would give and give and look at us kids with such pity and sadness. I hated going and seeing them at these churches and shelters. Free this and free that, they would brag and brag about how all this is fine and free, why work and try to do extra. "I do not need all of that crap those rich people want; I'm fine living this way." My mother was able to do more and just did not want to try. They would talk about all of the places they could go and all of the things they could do without having to pay for any of it. All they wanted to do was get drunk or get high on whatever anyone had so they would not feel how they felt about themself.

She was pushed and overworked as a child and lost her father at a young age. Her mother did not reason with her daughter and wanted her to not talk about her father, so the child harbors a trauma she had from the loss of her father. The pity she received form everyone around at the time was given to her to take time to heal. She was not allowed to love her father and miss him since her mother hated him for leaving her for another. She would live with this energy and pain from how her mother feels seeing her as an everyday reminder. Just one of the traumas from her life and realizing now how much different each trauma unresolved can add to the layers of one's unique complexity.

This is one of the reasons she would live in this fantasy and I could see her live in her mind and not knowing where she was. Swaying back and forth and daydreaming about the past and what happened all those years ago. She would tell stories about how she misses him and all the time she did not get how her mother would treat her and her sister differently and why she will never live like her mother. She would cry every time anything would trigger her about her father and would go right back into story, living in the past. She would not see where she was and what was going on. She had three kids to take care of. Living in the past numbing from the pain with substances and wanting pity from everyone around. Free food to live on in the spring, summer, and fall. Look for a place to stay over winter with people or in sheds and barns.

Having a home or a shelter was only during the cold season, so I spent more time out there than in a home with electricity and hot water. During these times on the river is where my heart still is.

The sound, the smell, and the beauty all around was so beautiful as the colors flow together. The sound of the river and feeling in the ground from the movement of the river and stone. If you stand bare foot on the edge of the river, you can feel the tumbling of a stone being moved with the river. I could tell the size from the times it would knock. The faster the knock the bigger the boulder. To stand and watch these rocks and stones be lifted and pushed like they were nothing. The power and awareness you need to have around water will keep you on your toes. You had to know the time of year you are in and what elevation you are at. If it were raining in the mountains to the north, you need to move camp back from water and make sure you don't have to cross any washes (river crossing) that could flood. Pay attention to the water level and always walk at least two steps away from edge. Water may have dug under the edge and will give out without warning. You can be trapped and held under by the falling dirt and stone, then drown.

Training here was so much fun learning from so many different people on the river and in the mountains. The stories and the knowledge I gained from the lessons I learned on the river would connect me to mother nature. I loved the outdoors and being in the mountains hearing and smelling the animals come and go. The sound of the trees whispering in the night while going to sleep. The birds chirping just before dawn. The soft steps of a black bear walking through camp while everyone sleeps, looking to get a free meal. Hearing the elk and deer crossing the river in the early morning hours. Waking up to having a herd of javelina (wild pig) in your camp and watching them move down river looking to cross. Mountain lions prowling the hillsides and watching you from the trees. The eyes in the night reflecting from the fire as they would come in to see what was going on. Bobcats playing in the evening running around chasing what they decided they wanted for dinner. Wolves would be around but kept their distance watching from across the river. When they would get close and try to surround the camp, we would all yell and make the fire as big as we could. Living so wild and being able to see nature and all her beauty in her natural state while being provided by the river with fresh spring water and food of all kinds. Rainbow trout and crawfish were always available if you knew where to look and fish.

I would use the heads of the fish I would catch putting them in a handmade twig basket to catch the crawfish. Place the basket in a shallow part of the stream and make it to where the crawfish would have to climb into the basket to eat of the head of the fish. Leave it there overnight and first thing in the morning, slowly walk to the basket. They can feel you walking from the sound of your movement next to the river. Slowly grab the basket and pull it up out of the water and see what you now have for brunch. Toss the crawfish into boiling water and wait until red hot and fully cooked. Tear in half and eat the tail then suck the juices out of the head. If you had butter you could tear the tails off and cook the meat in butter on the fire.

Fishing was easy and always a good idea when hungry. Start a fire and find a large stone that is flat on one side. Place on the fire with the flat side up so the stone heats up like a skillet. When you catch a fish, you can clean and scale it right there on the river attracting more crawfish for the evening trap. Place fish on the hot stone and flip using the tail. Once the bones and the tail pull away from the meat you can enjoy right there on the river's edge.

Now I know this may sound awesome, as well as scary, and everyone sees it for what it is. I loved this life, this place, and all the training I was able to receive during my first time on the river. Here I would be able to run and play and meet new people making friends while they were around. In town, people knew me and the family I was with but, on the river, I was able to be someone else for the time being.

I would sneak into other campsites up and down river and see how close I could get without being seen. Sometimes while they would be asleep, I would sneak over and steal food from other coolers, prizes like hot dogs, cupcakes, lunch meat, and whatever else my new neighbors would bring with them. They were such great neighbors. If I were ever seen, I would say I am sorry, I was trying to go around to our campsite down there, I am on way back to mine. Act innocent and just keep moving and they always just told me to be careful on my way. Such great neighbors.

I would teach some kids what I would do in the woods tracking and fishing in the river. If they could play since we had a reputation, I would get to meet new kids. While I lived there so many kids and families would all come and go. Girls would have fun teasing me for being a wild boy and boys wanted me to show them how to be wild. Make a spear and fish with it, or tie a rope around my waist, then tie the other end to a stick or stone and throw it over a branch. I would pull myself up to trees we could not climb before and is a good quick get up and away in a hurry if you need to get to high ground. Other kids thought I was so cool, or they thought I was scary as hell and did not like me. All I did was be myself and do what all I needed to do to survive and learn how to pay attention to more details in your surroundings.

I would look for the 'flat landers' we would call them; they are from the city or a different state. New tents and camper come with a shower, "Look at them folks and all their fancy shit," the men around me would point and laugh, and make people mad about having nice new things. They would talk down to people and make many uncomfortable and sometimes they would move to a new campsite. They did not like company, but I loved new friends and would go to find them to see. At night I would fly through the woods and form shadow to shadow. Slide to the side and looked through the coolers and boxes. Take what had double or looked like they had much of, I would just take for me. The next day I could walk the river and they would ask me to dinner if one of their kids wanted me over. They would ask all these question about why we live here, and I would tell them it's all we can afford. The looks on their faces and the way they would think of me living this life would flash in their minds. They would give what they could, and they would sometimes give hope, and some would ask me to go away. They were not comfortable with their kids playing with a homeless boy on the river. I never took offense, nor did I ever cry about being treated like I was. It was a good reminder that even people with money had their own hate and ignorance.

I did however take more from the ones who treated me like a wild animal. Like the ones who told me to get out, and get back, or go to my tent. Like I was a dog and supposed to run back to my house and hide. I would look at them and grin and say okay, have a good night. In my mind, *I'll be back and I have already memorized your supply*. I would not tell the men in my camp for this flatlander would die so I would never get them involved. This is my river and you are in my home. Yes, I am small, but dangerous, nevertheless. I took more than I should and the next morning we heard the man asking about his cooler. He was laughed at by the others and told to drive back home and get more.

I thought it was funny until I seen the kids with them were sad and it ruined their trip. No longer did I like what I did. They stayed anyway and had enough still, they been just mad at what happened. I would go by late at night and hear the man yelling and the kids and the mother sitting there quietly looking sad. I could see no matter the money life was not always what it seemed. The stories from the kids I would meet and things I would see and how so many had their own struggle. Though in a way it was different from mine, but the life was what we are raised by. Hateful father or a drunk of a mother or choose the whole latter for fair sport.

There were different rules on the river but, the same sexual encounters would run free in the woods as well. Young girls and boys, and girls and girls, I would see and be asked to join. We all were learning and liked to play but the rules are all the same. You must both agree to play and then we would find out and see what each other liked and wanted to try. We learned from the sounds and the stories we heard from the other parents and what we hear in our own homes. When you are in the dead of night and the sound is clear and then begins a moans and noises. Bite it and smack that, pinch them harder we would be listening to the banter. Sometimes the noises they would make huffing and puffing, and grunting would make you laugh. I would try not to and hold it in but, sometimes it was just too funny. If some started early and the smacking would start, we would make noises and laugh at them while they were in the tent or behind the trees.

No one ever minded and open we all were it was natural and exciting to have sex in the wild. So, of course the young would see and find out about it when no one was around to see. While the adults run to town and us kids watched the camp, we had so much time to play. Many questions and lessons the boys and girls learned and we caught on quick. Each one of my sister's friends I have seen naked and have played with.

It was not weird to us because we would sometimes bathe together. When you wash in the river and do not have a bathroom you will become one with nature. Naked in the mountains I would dry in the sun against a warm boulder raised out of the river where we would bathe. Quite a few times I would see girls and others see me and watch me from the banks of the river. Love for one another with life and beauty all around will captivate you. I will just say there was not a question to age or morals in those hills. If you both knew and wanted to play, they would do so when no one knows. At the drop of a hat you could get called to a tent and from there the story goes. I know you want it, and here it is you have no time to think this through. I want it now and you will do, hear I'll take it from here the woman or girl would tell me.

I could feel the energy of excitement and fear of the unknown as well as the thrill of doing something so wrong from today's societal standards. I would be used for pleasure and curiosity learning to deal with hormones and taboo. Some of the older girls would use me to stimulate the energy for what they were calling in and wanted to create. Spells and enchantment where the reason for a lot of the energy and I was shown how to stimulate a girl and what works best.

This training was for me to learn how to work female energy and how my sexual energy was stronger than most. I was told it was fascinating how I was able to be sexually active at this age and that I fully understood what I was doing. They would make me feel like I was incredible and was proud of this energy I have and can share with others. Now I understand the reason for all the love and the sex others would use to feel better. Coming from a place like I have it was the only way to feel the way it makes you feel when you are together sharing lust and passion. Forgetting about the pain and darkness we are surrounded by and live through every day.

Homeless with no schooling or support that we can receive due to the adults we belong to. Never told we are capable and able to have anything we want and can be anything we want to be. Not allowed to say, "I love you," get a good night kiss or tucked into bed. No hugs and love shared when you learned something new or if you did something you were proud of. You would hear, "Get the hell out of the way, I don't care." Told you were nothing and will never succeed and you're doomed before you even started on your life. Not just the children or the teenagers but the parents raising us as well. They lived through similar or maybe worse, but I know I could feel the desperation to feel pleasure over pain. How they would moan and scream and just ask to make them feel better sometimes alone and afraid of the shadows behind them. What they needed I could see, but I could not provide what they needed; I was just a boy at the time.

Taboo and wrongdoing made it more thrilling and they would want and crave more. From the woods to a tent and sometimes a vehicle thing would happen anywhere you can go. The men would take girls out to the woods and sometimes to town or so we were told. We would be hunted and stalked as in the wild like prey to a predator, the women and girls would lust for sexual conduct. Love was learned and lust was a way to enjoy all who you encounter. Some mothers would tell the young girls to go and play with him he is cute, and I would just take you home with me if I could. Wanted me to kiss their daughters and would talk openly about how young she was when she started to play with boys and what she did. Stories about men and women now and how we should all love open and explore one another.

The witches along the river and in town loved to enchant and threaten us young boys to watch out. How they would drink our souls and break our bones if they were to give us a riding. They loved to play around and show their breast, showing me that they wore no panties. Showing me how to touch and where to lick on a women's skin and body. What girls like and what they all want and what real women will do to young men.

I can say I was happy to be in the woods where I could run and get away. I could meet new people and make new friends and was loved by so many. I was happy to be wanted and used if you will but, at least I felt no pain at the time. I felt wanted and loved and stimulated by touch, of the delicious smell of desire. I got to a point I could see what they wanted and without as much as a look. Sisters and mothers, and girlfriends of brothers, so many that love would flow. What we all wanted in the end was to feel pleasure and love while surrounded by this day to day pain and sorrow. I see now in the faces I remember and the pain they must have felt or gone through. What could have happened to this mother of many that gets excited from the power of seduction and taboo. While embracing the sensual pleasure of my soul's energy the girls would tell me I was special. Women were not so lucky and treated dirty and like they are less than a dog. The pain and fear for the sisters I had here, the girls of others in the same crew. Whatever they needed from me, I would be open to share, if it were love and passion to help see how they were loved and deserve so much more, then so be it.

I ask you to understand if you do not relate, or able to see the harsh reality of the world we see, and life we received as children with no choice at the time. We only knew what we learned from parents who taught use nothing but hate and ignorance and to take all you can before you die. No one wanted to help, and everyone hated us for where we are from. They would teach that we only have each other and to never turn your back on family. Family is not your blood and not your last name. It was the ones you hold closest to your heart and who is there for you at your darkest times. Brother or sister was just a word to describe your gender and not your blood status or relations. Others would say no way and that does not happen.

It is okay you do not want to acknowledge and accept that this happens, and it is where you are supposed to be. Things happen to us for a reason and I was not going to let someone else's fear and taught hate effect the love I wanted to share. If you get the chance to love in the worst and hardest times, do it and embrace it. Never may you know this person again or ever watch this person grow but if you feel the connection then we would accept nature and love as we could.

Never did I force anything on any girl. Yes, I was taken advantage of as a young boy but, there was no one to tell and who would have believed me? Boys never tell when a woman takes advantage of them and uses you for sexual desires. Your brothers would tell, and the sisters would cause trouble if they knew you played with their mother. So, it was wise to keep quiet and to myself.

I would live like this for a while and the nights started getting colder and colder. Winter was moving in and new neighbors came less and less each weekend. I started to tell the feelings were now getting more and more of what to do and what we needed to do hearing winter was coming and it was time to go. They would leave me in the woods sometimes days on end and I oversaw the camp. I would get the firewood and clean up the camp burning all paper, plastic, and trash. No trash left behind, and I would watch to make sure everyone was safe from what was lurking in the shadows.

It was one of those nights I remember the sight of the eyes of a mountain lion watching me. First flash from a glare from the corner of my eye, late in the night as I started to fall asleep. I awoke to the noise of a low rumble and thought it was from the truck down the way. Where are they going this late at night? I poked my head out to see what is going on. It was not the engine but the sound of the lion's growl. I saw the back half of the lion walk next to the tent where my mother was sleeping. What a rush to see this wild animal around me I want to see him, but I know this could get violent. I grabbed my knife and my spear by my side I was going to challenge this monster to leave. Out of the tent I rushed straight to the fire and tossed four logs on the pile. As the light grew and the shadows got replaced with the light of the fire. I walked to my mother's tent where the lion was and looked around the tent. Nothing there and nothing to be seen so I quickly turned my back to the tent and kept my guard up preparing for battle. Look where he is and listen for him, or you could be his midnight snack. I was totally focused and played out in my head how I would use my spear first to defend. If I had to throw the spear to remember to keep my knife in my weak hand so I could grab the lion's neck to keep him from biting me and with my right hand, I would stab over and over. Grab the neck and rise it up all you can to keep from getting bit. They kill from above and smother your face or lock on to your neck. I was exposed and not able to see where the lion went but I knew to stand with my back to the fire. They were afraid of the fire and I was ready for a head on attack. I looked to the trees and nothing to see, no eye shine or even a glow. I waited all night until, first sight, of the sun coming up over the mountains as it glowed. I placed a couple logs and went to my tent and slept for just a few hours. After getting up and checking and looking for tracks I could see what he did during the night. He came down the mountain and circled my tent twice. Moved through the camp searching and tracking where we all walked. He tracked the fish to the camp from the smell of the fish we caught and cleaned on the riverbank. When I tracked him to where I had seen him by my mother's tent. The tracks were gone, and I was confused for the track looked like they went into the tent. No others around and I did not know how the lion would disappear like he did. All I could think of, is that he must have climbed the trees. By the time I came out he must have run out and disappeared while I was guarding the camp.

Quite a few times me and this lion would cross paths. There was once I caught him tracking me as I was tracking him. I was following his trail up the mountain and it was getting late. On my way down I realized at the base his tracks were doubled back and somehow behind me, but I did not see him on the ground. So, as I walked back to the camp, I must have walked under him while he was in a tree. So, conflicted I was to how this animal would be so close but always able to evade me. I would sit and listen at night and wait for the rumble or growl. I would prepare all I could and wanted to see this beauty of a beast most would see as a monster or violent. I knew he was simply curious and wanted to see just who we are on his path for in the fall they move more south. Another night, a black bear moved through our camp. They have very distinctive sound they make while smelling and grunting to each other. If you do not have a bull horn or a gun to make a loud noise you must let them leave or make so much noise they run away. It is simple. If you freeze in fear you can die scared. If you use your fear to survive you will scare off anything in your camp. Unless it is a grizzly or large brown bear and your scare him first. If you come across wolves, you better have a way up a tree and wait for them to leave or a way to hurt the alpha. That is why I would also have two large rocks I would keep in my tent so I could smack them together to make the sound of a gun going off to make them run back to the mountains. Waking the others yelling wolf or bear, everyone knew to make noise, clap, or scream, and they would retreat to the woods.

During this time, I spent on the river only once did I have Bigfoot up close and checking me out. I was sleeping in my two-man tent and awoke from the sound of someone walking around through the brush. I woke up and was listening to heavy breathing and heavy steps across the sand on the back side of the camp were my tent was. Waiting and listening and wanting to know what it was or if it was one of the crew looking for a place to pitch a tent or to just sleep. Sometimes it was the sheriff or rangers walking through checking for drugs, narcotics, paraphernalia, or whatever they wanted to check for. I could always tell when it was one of them from the way they would walk quickly and steady. Swift movement and the sound of the clothes they wore. The outfit they wear makes a distinctive sound when the pants and shirt rub together from walking.

As I lay there listening someone walked to my tent and pushed down on the top of my tent and fingers dragged down the side making the sound of sliding nylon across your fingers. The growl after that was not a man or a bear, this was deeper, and you could feel the energy in the area shift. A sense of fear and silence followed. The smell of moss-covered trees roots on the river came into my tent and it was extraordinarily strong. Just then someone got out of their tent and walked to the tree line to relive himself of his alcoholic beverage from earlier. He mumbled a few things and made a relief sound and stumbled back to the tent and back to sleep. I heard nothing more or after that until the bird's chirping welcoming mornings approaching.

After everyone awoke, I asked if anyone seen or heard what

happened. I told everyone what was in the camp and asked if anyone seen or heard anything? I started looking for tracks and the men helped to see if it was the law moving in on us and checking to see if we had to move deeper into the mountains upriver. The tracks in the sand was like a man's but larger. I asked my mother's boyfriend if it was him who got up last night and if he saw anything. He said he thought he saw someone walking through the camp. He asked who they were with no response, so he said I thought he was seeing shadows because it did not move or make a sound. He went back to bed and thought nothing of it.

I told them what happened, and they looked at the prints and flowed them all over the camp. Big foot they said asking again what all I remember and if he thought it was a man or a bear double stepping. If the back-paw lands with the front paw print as the bear walks, it can look like one large print. He said you know what? I remember thinking he was too tall and wide to be a man but since he was drunk, he said I really did not care. I thought it was a tree and if it was not and he did nothing to me then I am not worried about Bigfoot being around. I do not want to hurt him so why would he hurt us? This is his home and if he does not want us here, he would let us know. He told me about the tree knocks and the screams we would hear down the canyons at night. Rocks being thrown into the river and trees being pushed over to the ground. Shelters they would find in the mountains and dead animals that had their necks broke and then eaten.

I started to pay more attention to the sounds in the distance and down the river. I felt so honored to be allowed to share this area with something so awesome and mystic. When he asked who is there and nothing responded he just said, "I was too tired to care." Now that he is thinking about it, he can see how the two would compare. We tracked him to water and the river was too deep to cross without a rope. We left it alone for what can you do but hope he just leaves you alone. Shortly after that we had to pack up and move back to town for winter was almost here.

We stayed with friends of my mothers and friends of the family constantly moving from place to place. We could wear out our welcome quickly due to the fact my mother and her boyfriend would fight and argue every night. They would cause issues and drama and be told or asked to leave and some of them had the police show up from fear of my mother's boyfriend telling them he would kill my mother, me, or someone in the place we were staying. When he got drunk, he got violent and wanted to fight or hurt someone. He would get drunk and leave and get caught stealing, fighting, running from the police, or warrants for child support.

I would get small breaks from him and every time my mother would take him back with open arms.

I liked the new places we would go because I would be able to learn more about anything the people, we would stay with knew about. Building things, making things, fixing things, I would watch and help all I could. I loved helping ranchers work the property learning irrigation and how to run water lines and how gravity worked forcing water to the animals. Checking on the food levels of the animals and cleaning up after them.

I like to do a good job and loved being told I was a good worker and helper. I would hang around the adults since not too many other kids could hang with me since I was my mother's bastard son. One place we stayed for a little while was outside of town called Upper Round Valley. My mother's boyfriend's grandmother lived out there in a nice home we would call a double wide trailer but to me it was a mansion. Large open property and plenty trees and bushes to play and hide in when I wanted to disappear.

It was another Christmas and they had everyone's kids over including my mother's boyfriend's children. We all slept in a room together and then we woke up to them saying Santa has come, so come on out and we all ran out to the living room. Everyone started getting handed present and then I realized I did not get anything. Nothing for me this year, I guess. I was told I should not have been bad and cause so much trouble and may be then I would get something next year.

I sat and watched everyone else get toys and games as well as clothes thinking one day, I will get something too. His grandmother went into her room and grabbed a pack of socks and walked them over to me. She told me, "Here take this, they were for a larger boy but you will grow." I was so happy to receive this gift, brand new socks! What a treat this was! I was wearing shoes without socks for a while and she gave me a pack of one of her boys. I will always have love for this grandmother for making me part of the Christmas I was left out of. I was so happy to have socks I popped a hole in the bag and put on the new pair just so I could sleep in them. My mother's boyfriend's daughter made me sleep with her that night. She held me and told me it will be okay, and she loved me no matter what. I will be fine and do not let anyone tell me different. She was the only one there who was nice to me. My own brother and sister still treated me as an outsider and called me a bastard, that I was not really their brother. A lot of people would have hate and jealousy about a lot of these situations but I could see they hated me for their own reasons and I decided to just pay attention to what I had to do until I could get out on my own.

TWENTY
PUMPKIN CENTER

The next place we lived was a town called Pumpkin Center on the edge of the Tonto Basin Native Reserve. It was a smaller town and we lived in a hotel from the start. I remember sitting outside at night when it was a coolest time with the night breeze over the desert basin and through the mountains. I tried to sleep outside or try to be away from inside the hotel as much as I could.

My mother and her boyfriend would have sex in front of us kids while trying to get to sleep. I was the smallest and I would sleep on the floor while my brother and sister shared the pullout sofa. He would get out of bed naked and walk to the bathroom stepping over me. I would just keep my eyes closed and try to stay quiet having to listen to what they did on the bed. She would do the same and had no problems with how things were going if she had beer and this man in her life.

I tried to make friends in the neighborhood, but things got a little difficult once people found out who I was and who I was with. We finally got a trailer to live in out of town in a small edition and I went to school there for a short time. The classes were different from most and the school was a small warehouse with no windows. Classes held multi grades in it like first through third grade and fourth through sixth and so on. I was able to meet new people, but I was poor, and people already knew I was a bastard child. Kids would tell me they were told not to talk to me or be friends. The only one I was able to see outside of school was the other bad kids that no one wanted around. I still had lice and so everyone was told to stay away and that I was not allowed to sit with other kids because I had lice. No playing with others or much talking to others since everyone was open about me living with lice.

What I remember most about this place was the darkness that came back into my life. I would stay outside most of the time since the adults would be inside drinking and partying. I would go on long walks through the basin tracking and following coyotes and bobcats. The night was my favorite for the stars would shine bright and I loved looking to the sky. Sometimes I would get so far out and lost in the sky I would lose track of time. Getting back as fast as I could so I would not get in trouble I would run and get into the trailer. Most of the time they did not know I was gone and tell me to go back outside if they did not want to see me inside. I would go back outside and sit on the trunk of the car we had outside leaning back on the windshield looking into the stars, getting lost on the colors of the sky.

I would dream about leaving and going out on my own living a different life than this. This was the place I remember the dreams that would wake everyone from my screams. I would dream about hearing my mother scream and I would walk into the kitchen and see a chair in the middle of the kitchen floor covered in blood. As I would try to get to my mother's room, I would sink into the blood on the floor up to my ankles and would get stuck unable to reach her door. I would try so hard to get to her I would fight and scream to the point of waking up screaming running to check on her. I would get in trouble and smacked for waking them up and told to stop crying and being a little bitch. She would tell me she was fine, and it was just a dream, but I still remember it clearly. Another dream I would have was I would walk out to the car to get in so she could take me to school and she would be dead in the driver's seat. When I would reach for her, I would be stuck and could not move to try to help bring her back to life. She was just sitting there dead lifeless and unresponsive. After I would wake up, I would go check on her and learned to check first and try not to wake anyone while I was checking on her. Other dreams were of creatures and animal like beings chasing me and taking me by the hand a leading me outside and pointing to the road. Sometimes I would be in bed and could not move seeing these shadows looking down at me. I could not fully see them, but I could see the eyes and the shape of the torso. If I tried to yell I could not, and I felt like something was sitting on my chest not allowing me to speak or to get help. After a while I would black out and wake up to morning with birds chirping and sun glowing. I could not tell if it was a dream or if it really happened. I stopped telling people what I was dreaming from the reactions I would get while telling the story. Shadows floating on the ceiling and standing in the corner watching me. I found it best to just keep all of this to myself. This was a place of struggle while living under the most beautiful night sky. I learned things like, if you drive a stick shift vehicle and you must pop the clutch of the engine by parking on a slant or have enough people to help push. You must know when you get to a new location you need to look for a place to park that has a slant to it so the car will move forward easily. Seven years young and this is what I learned by watching. Asking questions got me into trouble so I just watched quietly and learned quickly.

Get inside the vehicle and depress the clutch to shift the car into 'Neutral'. Insert the key into the ignition and turn it to the 'On' position. This is the place the key would be after a normal turn of the ignition switch for starting. Instead, with a clutch pop, the ignition will already need to be on so that when the engine is turned over, the key is in the on position. Move the car in position to be pushed from behind or sent down a slope for the starting procedure. When in gear, the engine will be forced to crank, and the ignition will send a spark for a start. The quicker the vehicle is going before the clutch is released will determine how many times the engine will turn over. More cranks equal more opportunities to ignite the gas and air for combustion and the engine to start without a battery or starter. This helped me want to learn about celestial mechanics, the branch of astronomy that deals with the motions of objects in outer space. Historically, celestial mechanics applies principles of physics (classical mechanics) to astronomical objects, such as stars and planets, to produce ephemeris data.

At only seven years young and still a lot to go through, I had the basic understanding that life has many different faces and personalities to deal with in a day. You are only what you can provide or keep up with along the way. If you fall behind, you will be left behind. Survival of the fittest and most feared by the area of the place you are in. Fear is what keeps you alive and what will take control away from others. Pain is essential to life to remind you that you are alive and not happy with the predicament you are in while un-happy. Go ahead and re-read that last line I know you will need to process it. I did when I wrote this. I've seen pain and suffering as a trial by fire so I will be accepted by the same men and women in my life treating me so bad. Not knowing there was another way or seeing a way out. This is the tactic of survival. You do not have to like it but you will act like you love it so you can eat with the pack and be accepted into the only family you have ever known. Hate was fuel for any revenge needed and stored in the body as a reserve so you could turn it on at any time. Fear was switched to reaction and no longer did any man scare me, I just knew what to do at all times to demobilize any size man in any situation with a long list of items that can be turned into a weapon.

Love was a word made up for fairy tales and love songs and has no real meaning in this society. Man likes women and women likes man, so if one craves the other, enjoy what this life has while in this short miserable painful experience; Or if one wants the other, the games and challenges are put to the test and by whatever they come up with. A need to fulfil the taboo or craving they have. It was like animals with societal habits and traditions testing one another and challenging for the titles they imagined they were fighting for. How they lived in the ideas they would create from stories they never actually heard. Like, the town really hated them, no one really liked them, and how everyone judges them and talks behind their backs. It was a life and reality that they as an individual would create a story of a family not liking them and talking about them, so they then wanted to rob them and rape the wife while the husband watched. I heard these words many times while seven years young and already trained how to kill someone in 0-15 minutes. I was also trained on how to get into any home, vehicle, and store, so I can open the door from the inside for whoever was part of the raid party (like Pirates). Stalking and tracking people without them knowing while moving in and out of shadows and cut throughs (alleys). Knowing how to tell where you are from the sun and stars with the cardinal directions and knowing where you are coming from. Mind and body connected from learning how to heal the body and focus on breath work. Witchcraft and Magic, Native dances and tantric, the list of experiences grows. Life in the mountains, shacks, tents and cabins, the night sky, the amazing glow.

Child energy absorption and programming happens when a child is raised in and with different frequencies and lifestyles. Like violence or high stress. Children feel more than they visually comprehend, so what the parents and close kin feel, project and emanate (of something abstract but perceptible) issue or spread out from (a source), the children absorb. The feelings are hate, sadness, pain, loneliness, depression, and anger. This will subconsciously program habits and reactions to relationships and life choices in the future. Emotional programming is how the body remembers and reflects the feelings you carry inside. The severity of the emotional programming will depend on how many traumas (a deeply distressing or disturbing experience) the individual holds in their body memory. Like the pain we have in our everyday life. Emotions can program the body to react in a craving or a physical pain depending how the individual has stored the information.

Understanding the emotions and the triggers that make us react and do the things we do, so we can acknowledge them. Once acknowledged and accepted as the past and choose to no longer let this situation effect our life, we can remove the old habit created when we did not understand. Simple innocent unknowing of the reality of the choice we make for our self every day. Emotional sensitivity refers to the ease or difficulty with which your children respond emotionally to various situations. This trait is measured on two scales. The first scale measures how tuned in your children are to their own feelings. Some children are overly sensitive emotionally to their own feelings and feel things very deeply, while others do not seem to be aware of what they are feeling at all. The second scale measures how sensitive your children are to others' feelings and emotions. Some children are very tuned in to what is going on for others and other children appear to be non-responsive to what they see emotionally around them. It is important to note that some children can be high on one scale of emotional sensitivity and low on the other. They may be very aware of their own feelings, even to the point of being self-absorbed, while not aware of other people's feelings, and vice versa. The brain changes that stress can cause are not only hormonal, they can also be genetic or 'epigenetic', which is a burgeoning area of research.

Epigenetics is the study of how genes can be turned on or off with certain environmental cues, stress being one of them. One study found that when parents are significantly stressed during their child's first few years of life, some of the children's genes – involved in insulin production and in brain development – were affected even years later, in adolescence. "This seems to be the first demonstration, using carefully collected longitudinal data, that parental adversity during a child's first years leads to discernible changes in his or her 'epigenome', measurable more than a decade later," said author Michael Kobor. "This literally provides a mechanism by which experiences 'get under the skin' to stay with us for a long time. Pregnancy isn't the only time that parental stress can affect the development of the offspring – the relationship continues right through childhood."

Animal studies have suggested similar ways in which maternal stress level can affect the offspring's behavior and ability to cope with stresses, right down to the genes. There is a famous series of experiments by Michael Meaney at McGill University, in which rat mothers with low stress levels, who spent a lot of time licking and grooming their pups, had pups who were calmer and more exploratory than rat pups who only got licked a little (there's a great synopsis of the studies here). And this difference lasted throughout the pup's lifetimes. But the most intriguing part is that the rat pups of 'minimal-licking' mothers who were then cross-fostered to 'frequent-licking' moms ended up with the behavioral makeup of their new foster moms. And amazingly, these differences went all the way down to the genes in rat pups' brains, with certain regions being activated or deactivated (again, epigenetics), depending on what kind of rearing they had. These changes in their brains, spanning the gamut from genes to behavior, seem to stick with the animals for life.

These findings led the researcher, Harlow, to make lots of conclusions about the nature of love, like, "Love is an emotion that does not need to be bottle- or spoon-fed," and, "Man cannot live by milk alone." Whether the experiments are about love at all – or whether they are about what the offspring 'read' in their mother's behavior – is the more important question. Code suggests the most critical thing that we can transmit to our kids is not our ever-present, undying love – it's actually to provide them with a sense of calm and the absence of stress, which he says may be more powerful than declarations of love. This is what will ultimately help their growing brains wire normally, without having to accommodate for some vague sense of impending danger as they develop, which may or may not exist. Look at the past as an opportunity to see the beliefs and feeling that could be some of the blocks that hold you back from not addressing habits created from childhood.

Understanding the third point of view of any situation and looking at it with no judgment or opinion. In third-person point of view, the narrator tells us about what is happening in the story. In third person, the narrator shows us the thoughts and feelings of one character. In third person, the narrator is all-knowing and shows us the inner world of every character that appears. If something is meant to be, it seems certain to happen, usually because it has been decided by God or other forces that people believe cannot be controlled. Stop questioning. Stop over-thinking. Stop looking back and trying to measure where you have been or how far you have left to go. Stop telling yourself you are not there yet or are not good enough. Thousands of moments led up to this. Hundreds of decisions and actions. Millions of tiny thoughts and mistakes and blessings have brought you here. For some reason we keep telling ourselves that we are not enough, that we have so far to go, that we will never reach this supposed 'level' or 'standard' we hold ourselves to. But we forget that every step of the journey is part of the journey. We forget that there are going to be rough patches on the road to success, that there will be downs to each of our ups, and that sometimes we are not going to be moving at all, but instead standing still. And all these places are okay. We are supposed to get tired. We are supposed to get stuck. We are supposed to get stagnant. Because these places are temporary and will eventually change. Just like we will have moments of great success, moments of absolute perfection, moments where we cannot stop smiling because it feels like everything is falling into place. See, everything is a part of the journey. Every high and low, good, and bad, moment of peace. We just must remind ourselves that we are doing fine—right where we are. We must tell ourselves that we are strong and capable, that we can push through whatever we decide to. You are where you are supposed to be and learning what you are meant to learn in the time you are supposed to learn it.

Learn what you need to and let the rest go. No matter how much structure we create in our lives, no matter how many good habits we build, there will always be things that we cannot control — and if we let them, these things can be a huge source of anger, frustration and stress. Realize that you cannot control everything. I think we all know this at some level, but the way we think, act, and feel many times contradicts this basic truth. We do not control the universe, and yet we seem to wish we could. All the wishful thinking will not make it so. You cannot even control everything within your own little sphere of influence — you can influence things, but many things are simply out of your control. There will be things that happen from time to time (someone's sick, accident happens, phone call comes at five a.m. that disrupts things, etc.) that will make you break your routine. First step is realizing that these things will happen. Not might happen but will.

There are things that we cannot control that will affect every aspect of our lives, and we must accept that, or we will constantly be frustrated. When you feel yourself getting angry or frustrated, take a deep breath. Take a few. This is an important step that allows you to calm down and do the rest of the things on this list. Practice this by itself and you will have come a long way already. It is important to realize that, just like when you learn any skill, you probably will not be good at this at first. Who is good when they are first learning to write, or read, or drive? No one I know. Skills come with practice. So, when you first learn to go with the flow, you will mess up. You will stumble and fall. That is okay — it is part of the process. Just keep practicing, and you will get the hang of it. It helps me to see things as funny, rather than frustrating. Car broke down in the middle of traffic and I have no cell phone or spare tire? Laugh at my own incompetence. Laugh at the absurdity of the situation. That requires a certain amount of detachment — you can laugh at the situation if you are above it, but not within it. And that detachment is a good thing. If you can learn to laugh at things, you have come a long way. Try laughing even if you do not think it is funny — it will most likely become funny.

When we get things the way we like them, we usually do not want them to change. But they will change. It is a fact of life. We cannot keep things the way we want them to be ... instead, it is better to learn to accept things as they are. Accept that the world is constantly changing, and we are a part of that change. Also, instead of wanting things to be 'perfect' (and what is perfect anyway?), we should accept that they will never be perfect, and we must accept good instead. Remember when I asked what 'perfect' is? Does perfect mean the ideal life and world that we have in our heads? Do we have an ideal that we try to make the world conform to? Because that will likely never happen. Instead, try seeing the world as perfect the way it is. It is messy, chaotic, painful, sad, dirty ... and completely perfect. The world is beautiful, just as it is. Life is not something static, but a flow of change, never staying the same, always getting messier and more chaotic, always beautiful. There is beauty in everything around us if we look at it as perfect.

Unleash the inner champion of your own story. We cannot all be elite athletes and champions, at least not in the traditional sense of competing at elite levels and winning medals. However, my belief is that there is a champion within each one of us and we can train like one at our own specific physical level. Regardless of what limitations you may have, there is a champion in you somewhere and it is simply a matter of finding that inner champion and unleashing him or her.

You can shatter your limitations, raise the bar on your performance and seek out and attain peak performance for each level of physical capability, you just must know how to begin. You must make the commitment and that comes when you set your goals. Training needs to be a major priority in your daily life or life will happen and throw you off the training track.

Commitment, you have set the plan, now work it. Training Consistency is an absolute key to the training regimen of any champion and that includes you. Over time, it is the consistency that pays off big dividends. Psychology trumps physiology and the mind connection to the body are huge when focusing upon positive results and outcomes. Visualize the win and because those champion athletes that visualize themselves winning, have a far better chance of winning than those that do not apply the head edge strategy.

Laser Focus – avoid distractions when training; put blinders on like a racehorse and concentrate on the road in front of you.

Keep your head and heart in the game. Do not focus upon obstacles. Believe in yourself because it is all about you at the finish line.

The Inner Champion is an aspect of the Self that supports us and helps us to feel better about ourselves. It encourages us to be who we truly are rather than fitting into the box our Inner Critic creates for us. It is a magic bullet for dealing with the negative impacts of your Inner Critic. One way to think about your Inner Champion is to see it as the ideal supportive parent that you always wished you had. It is an aspect of the Self that responds in a helpful way to Inner Critic messages. It helps you to see the positive truth about yourself instead of the negative lies from the Inner Critic.

In the face of a Perfectionist Critic, your Inner Champion supports your right to not be perfect. It reminds you that it is only human to make mistakes and that making an error does not mean there is anything wrong with you. It reminds you that you are totally okay even if you don't get everything right. It supports your right to have balance in your life— to rest, take care of yourself, and enjoy life. It knows that many jobs just need to be done well enough, not to super-high standards. It has the wisdom to know that sometimes it is important to go with the flow and let things evolve rather than trying to get everything perfect right away. It supports you in being a learner who does not have to know everything to start with. It knows the meaning of 'rough draft'.

An Inner Controller Critic judges you harshly to try to stop you from overeating, using drugs, or indulging in other dangerous substances or activities. In response, your Champion tells you that your real needs and desires are okay and that you are fine just as you are. It supports you in being relaxed and trusting your decisions about what you eat or what you do. It also supports you in being centered and in touch with your body, which naturally brings moderation. It supports your capacity for healthy pleasure and sensuality in life, which is satisfying enough that there is no need for overindulgence.

In the face of a Destroyer Critic, your Inner Champion affirms that you have the right to exist. It confirms that existence is your birthright. Your Inner Champion loves you and cares for you. It has great compassion for your suffering and wants you to feel good and whole. It holds you close and tells you that you are precious. This Champion nurtures you in the most fundamental bodily way, not only because you need it, but also because it loves to be close to you. Sometimes the Destroyer Critic turns anger or aggression inward; it turns anger toward you that was originally meant for other people in the outside world. Your Inner Champion can redirect that anger toward where it belongs. It affirms that you have the right to be angry with people who have hurt you or neglected you. It also tells you that you have the right to set limits, to protect yourself, or to be powerful—and yes, these may involve ending a job or relationship that is not right for you.

These descriptions are intended to inspire you and offer possibilities, not to limit or define your experience. Feel free to allow your Champion to emerge in whatever way is unique to you. All our Inner Critics are unique. You might have an Inner Critic that has characteristics of two of the described types or wants to be a called a different name.

A powerful antidote to the harsh and shaming Inner Critic voice is to develop an Inner Champion. The Champion does not try to argue or fight with the Critic or try to get rid of it. It supports us in being ourselves and in feeling good about ourselves. The Inner Champion is the ideal supportive parent. It helps us to see the positive truth about ourselves. It nurtures and cares for us. The Inner Champion helps us by setting boundaries with the Inner Critic, nurturing, providing guidance and planning actions.

Are you ready to Awaken Your inner Champion?

AUTHOR NOTE

I have always dreamed of telling my story, although for many different reasons over the years, the main gist was always the same. Circumstance is irrelevant; what matters is how you let it define you. But it was not until I embarked on a deeper healing journey that this dream of sharing my story was able to manifest into reality. Through the healing journey the dream turned into a passion and a must. I must share this knowledge with everyone who is ready to hear so they too could Become the Champion.

Thank you for taking the time to and opportunity to reset your beliefs, perspective, and story. Everyone has an inner champion; that winner that overcomes struggle and adversity. In 'Becoming the Champion' you not only choose to overcome adversity but to release the perspective of the past and future story. We all have the choice to remain in our patterns and be the victim of our story or 'Become the Champion'.

ABOUT THE AUTHOR

Korey Carpenter is a multifaceted healer, Certified Quantum Healing Practitioner and Life Coach. He is the founder of Korey Carpenter Ascension. He has reached the lives of tens of thousands of people with his message, mostly through podcasts and interviews and looks forward to reaching thousands more through his books, programs, and articles. At the time of creation for this book, he lives in Indiana but loves to 'move around' with his wife, Ani and daughter, Nala. However, he considers Arizona home.

www.ingramcontent.com/pod-product-compliance
Lightning Source LLC
Chambersburg PA
CBHW030439010526
44118CB00011B/713